Surviving
Medical
School

For David Jeremy, and Miranda

Surviving Medical School

Robert Holman Coombs

Insights commentaries by
Bernard Virshup

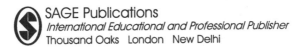

SAGE Publications
International Educational and Professional Publisher
Thousand Oaks London New Delhi

For information:

SAGE Publications, Inc.
2455 Teller Road
Thousand Oaks, California 91320
E-mail: order@sagepub.com

SAGE Publications Ltd.
6 Bonhill Street
London EC2A 4PU
United Kingdom

SAGE Publications India Pvt. Ltd.
M-32 Market
Greater Kailash I
New Delhi 110 048 India

Printed in the United States of America

Library of Congress Cataloging-in-Publication Data

Coombs, Robert Holman.
    Surviving medical school / by Robert Holman Coombs.
      p. cm.
    Includes bibliographical references and index.
    ISBN 0-7619-0528-6 (cloth: acid-free paper)
    ISBN 0-7619-0529-4 (pbk.: acid-free paper)
    1. Medical students—Life skills guides. 2. Medical education—
Psychological aspects. 3. Success. I. Title.
    R737.C66 1998
    610′.71′1—dc21   97-33951

98 99 00 01 02 03 04 7 6 5 4 3 2 1

Acquiring Editor:	Daniel Ruth
Editorial Assistant:	Anna Howland
Production Editor:	Michele Lingre
Production Assistant:	Karen Wiley
Typesetter:	Christina M. Hill
Cover Designer:	Kristi White
Print Buyer:	Anna Chin

Contents

Preface and Acknowledgments

If you were to climb Mt. Everest or any other challenging peak, you would do well to prepare by developing accurate expectations about the climb. Clear expectations, based on the experiences of others who have reached the summit, provide the best survival strategy. No matter what other coping skills you may have, if your expectations are not grounded in reality you will struggle unnecessarily.

Medical school and postgraduate training, not unlike mountain climbing, will require all of your inner strength and determination. Prepare now for the "climb" that lies ahead. Many students become discouraged, depressed, or drug dependent. Anticipate the challenges and vicissitudes so you will know what to do when you encounter them along your way.

This book is based on in-depth interviews with medical students at various stages of training. It also draws on my informal associations with medical students while chairing the Student Affairs Committee at the UCLA School of Medicine. Over the years, we implemented more than 20 well-being programs to benefit medical students. I have also drawn on my earlier publications that deal with physician socialization.[1-12]

I gratefully acknowledge the following medical students and physician colleagues who contributed to this book, as well as the students who participated anonymously: Andy Aligne, Kevin Armstrong, Debra Balke,

Martha Brewer, Vanessa Brown, Lilly Chen, Swayne Cofield, Lauren Crosby, Kerry Corboy, Gino Della Maggiore, Lien Do, Marc Feinstein, Jean Foreman, Beatrice Germain, Deborah Ginsburg, David Goldman, Maria Gonzalez, Stuart Hagen, Risa Joffman, Payam Kashfian, Jim Keany, Cynthia Kline, Mark Knoble, Dee M. L'Archeveque, Jerry Lipshulz, Alina Lupo, Tomoko Nakawatase, Jennifer Narcisse, Lily Nguyen, Thuong Nguyen, Quynh Giao Pham, Kris Potter, Jennifer Reifel, Kevin Rich, Sanjay Saint, Jared Salvo, Michele Saunders, Scott Saunders, Alison Savitz, Ira Smalberg, Alicia Starr, Gregory Stearns, Darryl B. Tam, Mike Ukeki, Rex Wong, Lance Wyatt, Edward Yu, and Ira Zunin.

JoAnn St. John, my co-author on a related book, provided insightful and colorful comments. Kate Coombs organized some of the material and contributed valuable ideas. Tiffany Tom, MD, and Suzanne Bovone improved the final manuscript.

I am very appreciative of the work of my beloved friend and colleague, Bernard Virshup, MD, who wrote the "Insights" section at the conclusion of each chapter. A medical humanist, he devoted his life to improving the lot of medical students. Bernie passed away just before this book went to press.

Finally, I express my deepest gratitude to Carla Cronkhite Vera and Carol Jean Coombs, who participated in every aspect of manuscript preparation. We have worked as a team on this project from beginning to end. Words cannot express my appreciation for their steady and productive work and enjoyable interactions.

Notes

1. *Mastering Medicine: Professional Socialization in Medical School.* New York: The Free Press, Macmillan, 1978.

2. *Making It in Medical School.* Jamaica, NY: Spectrum Publications Medical and Scientific Books, 1979.

3. *Inside Doctoring: Stages and Outcomes in the Professional Development of Physicians.* New York: Praeger, 1986.

4. *Drug-Impaired Professionals.* Cambridge, MA: Harvard University Press, 1997.

5. "Medical Marriage as Prevention for Physician Impairment." 1982, July-August. *California Academy of Family Practitioners,* 33(4):14-18.

6. "The Effect of Marital Status on Stress in Medical School." 1982, November. *American Journal of Psychiatry,* 139(11):1490-1493.

7. "Is Premedical Education Dehumanizing?" 1990, Spring. *Journal of Medical Humanities,* 11(1):13-22.

8. "Primary Prevention of Emotional Impairment Among Medical Trainees." 1990. *Academic Medicine: Journal of the Association of American Medical Colleges,* 65:567-581.

9. "The Primary Prevention of Addiction in the Physician." 1993. *Journal of Primary Prevention,* 14(1):27-47.

10. "Enhancing the Psychological Health of Medical Students: The Student Well-Being Committee" (Special Issue on Medical Student Well-Being). 1994. *Medical Education,* 28:47-54.

11. "Addicted Health Professionals." 1996. *Journal of Substance Misuse,* 1:187-194.

12. "The Impaired Physician Syndrome: A Developmental Perspective." 1986. In Cynthia Scott and Joanne Hawk, eds., *Heal Thyself: The Health of Health Professionals* (pp. 44-55). New York: Brunner/Mazel.

CHAPTER 1

Anticipation

Are My Expectations Realistic?

I came here thinking, "Doctors are Greek gods who never make mistakes and who heal—really cure the sick." One of the biggest hang-ups I've had is trying to accept what the doctor really is.

—First-year medical student

FRANK & ERNEST

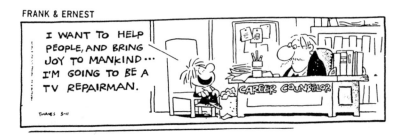

Typical premed students are academically strong and independent-minded. As a premed student, you were probably regarded by others—and even by yourself—as being the brightest and the best. "I have a high image of my intelligence and ability to do things," said an entering medical student. If you enjoyed this lofty position and took it for granted throughout high school and college, you are in for a particularly nasty shock when you start medical school.

Whether you are a student superstar or not, whether medicine is the only career you've ever considered or is a recent interest, formal training will probably not match your expectations. And you will probably conform to a far greater extent than you now believe possible to expected medical student behavior. As an individual accustomed to asserting your own outstanding abilities and expressing yourself independently, you may find this prediction unwelcome and largely unacceptable. And yet, it closely reflects the actuality of life in medical school as perceived by students who have experienced it:

> This is soooo true. It's like being in elementary school again. I remember at the beginning of my first year how it upset me that we all did every-thing together, including walking up and down the seven flights of stairs to and from class every morning and afternoon. I really felt like I had lost my individuality and become one of the 120 sheep in a flock. This was perhaps the most difficult part of my transition to medical school.

In the following chapters, you'll probably see your own interests, atti-tudes, and expectations reflected in the student comments that are quoted. These students' experiences may help you anticipate, understand, and accept the reality that awaits you.

The Premed Syndrome

In its most stereotypical and extreme form, *premed syndrome* describes stu-dents whose medical career goal dominates their lives. In their zeal to win the admissions race, these undergrad students—sometimes known as "gunners," "cutthroats," or "red hots"—sabotage lab experiments, conceal needed mate-rials from other students, and cheat on exams. The term describes those stu-dents who carefully select courses on the basis of the grades they can earn, perhaps avoiding otherwise attractive electives; who concentrate on their undergraduate studies with a uniquely fierce sense of urgency; and who or-chestrate extracurricular activities primarily with an eye toward impressing admissions committees.

Students may adopt specific premed syndrome behaviors because they feel they have little other choice: "I, too, have fallen into the trap of not taking the courses I'm interested in so I can fulfill my premed requirements," one said. "I was so concerned that I just avoided the classes whose GEs [general education requirements] I had already filled even though they sounded like I'd enjoy them more." Unfortunately, the premed syndrome is isolating. Other medical students, the only people who understand the extent of the pressure, may be regarded not as comrades but as threatening competitors. Everyone else is outside the experience, as one student observed: "My parents do not fully understand the rigors and stress involved even at the premed level no matter how hard I try to explain it to them."

The competitive behavior of relatively few students reinforces the concept of a premed syndrome: "When I was taking the lower division 'weeder' courses, the die-hard premed students who took them just because they were required were a lot less friendly than other people." "When it was time to interview, no one would share their experiences or give advice. I pretty much went through the process alone and blinded."

Confronting the syndrome stereotype can be trying for an altruistic student. "Throughout my undergraduate education," a premed recounted,

> I've been against the competition-focused mentality of the curve-graded premed classes. I've always gathered together study groups, held review sessions, and shared even my much-labored summary notes with my classmates. I've made some truly good friends who will be friends for life. But I've also been used many times over by classmates who only called when they needed help; they didn't associate with me once the class was over.

However individual students choose to handle it, the intense pressure and premature specialization among premedical undergraduates is real, as Karen Axelsson, older than her classmates, explains:

> Premed was a combination of nightmare and triumph. Always in the background was the anxiety that all this was only to apply, with no guarantees of acceptance. . . . Since my eventual selection from among tens of thousands of applicants seemed so remote, I focused on shorter term goals, doing the best I could in every class. I went at my studies with unprecedented vengeance. Whenever my motivation or energy started to founder, I imagined not getting into school and how I would feel if I had to attribute this to my own mediocre effort. Needless to say, the distractions of the moment just never seemed worth it.[1]

Earning the qualifying grades in required premed courses can become overwhelming and potentially life altering. Axelsson describes one such infamous premed course, organic chemistry:

> The two hundred and fifty-odd freshman and I were all united in our apprehension as the professor sailed blithely into his initial lecture on this terrifying and mysteriously important subject. Years of familiarity with the area had obscured his sense of how to make this material intelligible

to neophytes, and it was not until months later that I finally grasped what all this fuss over carbon was about.

During the first midterm, the tension in the lecture hall was palpable. There was not enough time to finish the examination, and when I got my test back several days later, I found I had gotten a 77—a solid C. I was undone. The small buds of confidence which had grown the previous quarter abruptly vanished, and utter failure and humiliation loomed on the horizon. I obsessed over the implications of this mediocre performance for the next week, breaking into tears every time I envisioned my dream slipping away. Finally, I realized that I could not afford to think about it any longer. Instead, I concentrated single-mindedly on mastering organic chemistry, studiously avoiding all thought of the future. Page by page, problem by problem, I forged ahead, cornering the head TA [teaching assistant] for hours each week to review problems and manipulate plastic hydrocarbon models with me.[2]

Many medical educators shrug off the premed syndrome as a natural offshoot of the intense competition to get into medical school, but others question the requirements and call for reform of the entire admissions process. At a meeting of the American Medical Student Association (AMSA), Dr. Bernie Siegel commented, "The applicant for admission to medical school is required to study chemistry, physics and biological sciences. Yet 90 percent of the activities of most physicians in daily practice require a philosophic or psychological approach. And I'd say also a spiritual approach."[3] Some reform has been considered and even tested on a limited basis. Nonetheless, medical admissions committee expectations send the traditional message: There is no substitute for a high grade point average and a record of excellence in the physical and biological sciences.

Expectations

Do you know what to expect in medical school? Surprisingly, even the most medically sophisticated students who come from "generations of doctors" seem to lack a clear perception of what medical training and practice will be like.

If someone had told me in advance what I would have to do, I would have said, "Forget it; it's not worth it to me." But once I was here and they handed me my ever-increasing stack of pharm cards, I thought there would be no way to learn them all in such intricate detail. Why couldn't I just look them up in a reference book? But to my amazement I did it! Med school is like that. They give you an impossible task and you do it.

Expectations About Medical School

The mystique of medicine is strong.[4] Many premed students romanticize physicians and their training. Everybody anticipates the cadaver experience in gross anatomy. Aside from that, student expectations range from a continuation of college—well understood and little feared—to an intensely grueling schedule that will require studying "all night every night."

Many students don't look beyond their goal to excel academically and gain acceptance to medical school. "I wasn't too sure of what the courses were going to be in the first year," one confessed. "I didn't even check into that." "I was afraid to learn too much in advance because it might discourage me too completely," said another. "I had so many reservations and concerns about entering the profession already."

Those who make an effort to anticipate the medical school experience still find surprises: "My image of what medical school would be like and what it is aren't the same!" "It's harder than I expected, more time consuming and demanding than I thought it would be." "I expected it to be hard, but I had no conception of how hard it really is."

A substantial number of first-year medical students are surprised and disappointed with the realities of medical school. Some cite the negative attitudes of faculty members toward them, the poor quality of instruction, lack of personal interest shown by the faculty, and the perceived irrelevance of the subject matter. If a general lesson can be drawn from their experiences, it is this: Be prepared! Learn as much as you can about what medical school is really like and adjust your expectations and behavior accordingly.

Expectations About Medical Practice

Interviewers at most medical schools asked you, "Why do you want to be a doctor?" If you could articulate your motivation then, remember it, because it's subject to change.

Career perceptions of entering first-year students differ markedly from those at later stages. Entering students, idealistic in their goals, usually stress the desire to serve humanity or to participate in a "breakthrough" to eliminate or control disease. They look forward to "helping people who need medical attention": "I've always liked to be around sick people and feel I can help them." "It is always good to be of service to people."

Science-oriented students may view medicine as an opportunity to "put the love of science to a practical use": "I can work with people and help them and still be involved with science." First-year students tend to glamorize physicians more than clinically experienced third- and fourth-year students. "I don't think there is anything about being a doctor that doesn't interest me," one said. "It seems like a good life that offers variety without boredom."

To a far greater extent than upper-division students, entering first-year students are almost apologetic about achieving a "better-than-average income." Nonetheless, visions of occupying a highly respected position drive them on: "Almost everyone thinks doctors are completely honest and have a high degree of integrity." "Everybody looks up to doctors." "I think it's probably the highest status position there is, the number one profession."

Some entering students formed their expectations by watching their physician family members—usually fathers—interact with patients and social acquaintances: "Seeing how people react to them influenced me to become a doctor." Others base their expectations on experiences as a patient or on television doctors: "I had asthma and had to see a doctor once or twice a week, and then my brother had corrective surgery from a condition that might have killed him. And my mother was also sick a lot. So family illnesses influenced my decision—and television reruns of Hawkeye Pierce, my favorite media doctor!"

Regardless of the source of their information, all students admire physicians for their intelligence, competence, and humanitarianism. "The most outstanding people I knew were in the medical profession," one said. "I know quite a few doctors at home. They just seemed like intelligent, knowledgeable people, and they impressed me. I guess I wanted to be like that too."

The greater an incoming student's romantic idealism, the greater the disillusionment about the real world of medical school, the teaching hospital, and future practice. In recent years the medical profession has come under scrutiny with the growing national health care crisis and malpractice lawsuits. "There's a lot of doctor bashing in the media." "Today's media docs are usually portrayed as greedy and insensitive, with only a few who can be changed to see the light."

Despite these frustrations, a medical career can be an exciting choice for those who come in with their eyes open; idealism needn't be entirely abandoned. A graduating senior explained, "The most valid reason for wanting to be an MD is still as true today as it was before—to help alleviate human suffering. The other reasons people give—prestige, money, independence— are all being whittled away by the changing economics of health care. I would have become a businessperson if I wanted those other things."

If you can accept potentially demoralizing experiences in your medical training; if you feel able to sustain your motivation and independence in the face of authoritarian attitudes and seemingly irrelevant academic drudgery; if your personal understanding of the physician's life goes beyond television's medical dramas, and this life remains appealing, then you are likely to enjoy medical school and the life of a physician.

Insights: Medicine and Stress
Bernard Virshup, MD

In my workshops on handling stress, I generally go around the room and ask each student to tell me a stress they are dealing with. We keep a list of these stresses. One such list recently read as follows: "Lack of time. Family responsibilities. Maintaining a healthy body. Not enough sleep. Fear of burnout. Living up to expectations. Balancing time between school, family, and self. Dating. Using time efficiently. Health. Eating a proper diet. Getting enough rest. Exam anxiety—can I learn it all? Lack of autonomy or freedom; loss of control. Fear of contracting an illness learned about in class. Fear of the future. Forming and maintaining relationships. Low self-esteem." Most medical students will relate to these. We could add many more.

What is stress? We usually perceive it as *external,* something that happens to us, from "out there"—situations, problems, events, people, deadlines, competition, examinations, critiques, time pressure, failures, mistakes, relationships. These can all be stressful but are only *experienced* as stress if they are internalized. Internal stress reactions are (a) uncomfortable emotions such as anxiety, fear, anger, frustration, helplessness, depression, shame, inadequacy, embarrassment, shyness, hurt, disappointment; and (b) uncomfortable physical reactions such as muscle tension, headaches, backaches, sweating, dry mouth, palpitations, high blood pressure, stomach cramps, nausea, diarrhea, insomnia.

How does *external* stress get converted to *internal* stress? Thoughts, beliefs, and perceptions, based on previous experiences, define the outside event or problem as dangerous or threatening. The threat rarely puts our lives at risk, yet it almost always threatens our self-image, our perceived worth. Much of what we experience as stress results from thoughts about ourselves that are actually irrational and untrue. And these can be changed!

The most common of these thoughts are

- It is terrible, horrible, and catastrophic when things are not going well. This is awful! I'll flunk! I'll starve! I could die! Nothing can save me!

- I should be more competent than I am. I'm not achieving enough. My worth as a person depends on how much I have accomplished and how well I am doing, and it's not good enough. I'm a fraud and a failure, and others are going to find out.

- I am selfish if I take care of myself. I will be a very good person and appreciated by others if I sacrifice myself for my career or for others.

- It is a dire necessity to be loved or approved of by almost everyone for almost everything I do. My worth as a person depends on how others see me and how much people like me or admire me. And if people knew what I'm really like, they wouldn't like me.

Where do these thoughts come from? Most psychologists think they are learned from parents who pay too much attention to accomplishments as a condition for approval. Rather than depending on *who they are,* approval is given to children based on *what they do.* Many medical students come from families in which to avoid parental displeasure or gain parental love they must prove their self-worth by constant accomplishments.

If you, like many students and physicians, have too large a conditional "if" to your self-esteem, then you are very vulnerable to the many stressors in medical training and practice. Now is a good time to reevaluate these beliefs. I, for one, believe that your value as a person is nonnegotiable and unconditional; it does not depend on what you accomplish. Think about it. What a difference such an attitude could make in your life. Instead of studying as a chore, study because you enjoy it. Instead of working for good grades, work because you enjoy what you are doing. Instead of working hard to gain someone else's approval, work because medicine is one of the most fascinating professions you could choose. Instead of worrying about what others think of you, become more interested in what you think of them.

If you do this, you will free yourself to take care of your own needs and prevent yourself from burning out. Those who constantly feel a need to prove themselves punish themselves by anxiously studying extra-long hours until they become inefficient and exhausted. They do so at their peril.

You need rest and recreation, good food eaten leisurely, good friends with whom you can exchange confidences and with whom you can spontaneously express your feelings. Take time to relax and enjoy the world.

Think about it, and take care of yourself.

Notes

1. Axelsson, Karen. 1986. "Pre-Med: A Personal Perspective." In Robert H. Coombs, D. Scott May, and Gary W. Small, eds. *Inside Doctoring: Stages and Outcomes in the Professional Development of Physicians* (pp. 12-18). New York: Praeger, p. 13.

2. *Ibid.,* p. 14.

3. Durso, Christopher, Laura Milam, and Molly Tschida. 1996, May-June. "Back in the Capital Again." *The New Physician,* pp. 27-34.

4. Barker, Debria A. Humphries. 1996, September. "Celluloid Doctors." *The New Physician,* p. 51.

CHAPTER 2

First Year

Am I Smart Enough?

My premed advisor used to tell me that premed classes like organic chem are used to separate men and women from boys and girls, and medical school simply turns those same men and women back into boys and girls.

—First-year medical student

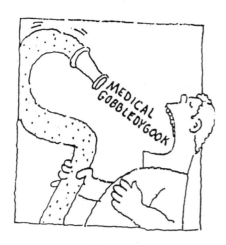

Idealistic beginners who dreamed of engaging in the war on disease while receiving stimulating on-the-job training at the hands of experienced clinicians often find themselves in lecture rooms and labs with unenthusiastic classmates eagerly looking forward to summer. Typical days consist of many hours of classroom instruction from a variety of research-oriented professors. "They lecture, you listen, then you go home to learn it on your own." "Living in the class-room with the same 144 students for two years—that was something I didn't anticipate." "The most frustrating thing for me is getting lost in lectures. If I get lost early on and stay that way for five minutes, then I'm washed up for the rest of the class. It's had a tremendous effect on me psychologically. I worry my classmates have been following the material and know what's going on." The frustration level intensifies when the course is not well organized:

Most students trust that our administrators and teachers know what they're doing, but they don't necessarily. For example, when they tried to revise our histology class they really messed up—it was very disorganized and confusing. We complained all semester about the class, but, amazingly, when it came time to do formal course evaluations, only 30 people filled out the forms. The faculty had to pester everyone to turn them in.

Not surprisingly, some disillusioned students begin to reassess their futures. "I held a lot of myths about medical school," one said. "I put doctors on a pedestal, thought they were the most intelligent, smartest, and all that. After being in school for a year and being jarred from a few of these myths, I'm seriously questioning whether it's all worth it."

Others are more sanguine. "Don't despair—the less-than-perfect system seems to work out in the end." "I look to some MDs and think, 'If that idiot can do it, *so can I!*'" "I know MDs aren't perfect. Med school was there for me to learn as much as I can so I won't make any mistakes as an M.D. I don't care how they teach it to me, just as long as they do." "They've been teaching it for years; if they think it's important or if it's discussed in detail in our text, I probably need to know it."

Workload

First-year students are often surprised and even overwhelmed by the academic workload. Although medical education can be improved in many ways, the volume of material to learn is inevitable. "Your behind takes the form of a chair."

It's not just the sheer volume of material to be learned, but also the unexpected—and unfamiliar—pressure to master course materials in a limited time. "It's like trying to drink from a fire hose," one student said. "It's impossible to learn everything put before you."

Fear of not keeping up is the principal source of stress for first-year students. "You may not think of yourself as the smartest human being in the world, but you think you are adequate. And then you get here and find you are inadequate. I'm becoming increasingly uncertain whether I should be in medical school." "I found it difficult to cope with the fact that I could study more than I'd ever studied before and still fail exams or do very poorly."

Previously high-achieving medical students face potential failure. "When I came here, I'd never had an F in my life. On my first exam in histology, I panicked, overlooked a page on the exam, and failed. I was shocked! To make up that grade, I stayed up all night before my first anatomy exam. The lab part was an hour and a half and the written part three and a half hours—I was so tired and drained I could hardly understand the questions I was reading. Well, I failed that one too."

Fear of failure engenders self-doubt and performance anxiety. "I was top in my class in high school, and in college I graduated summa cum laude. In the middle of my first semester, I was barely passing. Is med school too big to handle? Am I smart enough?"

> I don't think there's been a single quiz I felt prepared for. I study three or four nights for every one, but then before the quiz I come to the conclusion that I don't know enough. You could study 24 hours a day and not get it done. You finish studying for one test and then have to start studying for another one.

"The first semester I was scared to death all the time. It was the most depressing three months of my life." "I had periods when I was so paralyzed with fear I couldn't study."

> Before my histo exam I went in to ask a few questions and ended up having a mini-emotional breakdown—tears and all. I asked if it was normal to be so anxious and he said "No!" I lost 10 pounds without trying. As it turned out, I scored in the high 90s. I can't tell you how many times I looked at that grade and wondered if it was a mistake; I was too afraid to ask about it. But it did give me confidence that I can do the work if I put the work in.

Even when students pass the tests and complete other measurable course requirements, they are unlikely to feel like academic all-stars, let alone future physicians:

> The student doesn't have enough time to learn it like he wants to. A lot of the material is crammed in and you just don't get a good foundation. You look back and see that it hasn't been anyone's fault but your own, but there is no way; you can't give up sleeping. But, oh, how you try!

Because of the sheer quantity of material, many students trudge through their course work with the sensation of barely surviving. This would be daunting in any discipline, but medical students tend to feel that the smallest gap in their knowledge could mean the death of some future patient. "I became emotional sometimes and would say, 'Damn this stuff' and try to move on to other material; I just couldn't spend any more time on it. That really bothered me because I kept wondering if it's really something that I need." "There's just too much material to learn thoroughly," another added, "and I'm reluctant to move on to new material with only a superficial understanding of the topic, and can only hope I'll have the opportunity later to learn it better."

Fortunately for most students, academic failure is a feared rather than an actual disaster. "Many of my friends—including myself—constantly talked of our fear of failing anatomy or histology first semester, but needless to say, none of us did." Eventually, most class members recognize that they are not alone in their feelings of frustration and inadequacy. Some achieve this understanding and adjustment independently; many others seek advice. "I went to see my adviser and he assured me that while my counterparts aren't saying much about it, they are doing roughly the same as I am. Thank goodness they are as scared as I am." "I found it helpful to study with friends in the class. It made me realize I wasn't the only one feeling overwhelmed by it all." "My first impression was that the other people in my class were highly intelligent, more intelligent than I'm finding out they really are. Now, I'm finding myself just as capable as any of them." "I've learned that everyone has their strengths and weaknesses and to not be intimidated by someone who can rattle off information. It just may be that they studied it the night before."

Most students gradually come to grips with the workload and realize the impossibility of assimilating everything. "You reach the point where the stress is beating you down. After this happens two or three times, you say, 'Wait a minute. I'm killing myself, I can't do it. I'll put in just so much effort, and that's all I can do without hurting myself.'" "I did a little better after I started saying I'd go to bed at a certain time each night instead of trying to learn a little bit extra. You can learn more in less time once you budget your time. If you try to learn it all, you wind up learning nothing." "It doesn't always mean extra study. Sometimes it means listening more effectively." "You don't spend a lot of time on nonessential assignments. It's useless unless you want to be number one or two in your class. Those people study everything!" "Being number one doesn't equal being the best physician. Those top people sometimes have no personal skills with patients."

Pressure to learn everything is often self-imposed. The dread of making an incorrect diagnosis, prescribing improperly, or otherwise harming a patient through ignorance or negligence is very real, and it persists throughout one's career. A saying at a midwestern medical school illustrates how these fears evolve; it goes like this:

Premed Student: "Am I going to get in?"

Freshman: "Am I going to make it?"

Sophomore: "Do I really want to do this?"

Junior: "Will I ever know enough?"

Senior: "Will I ever know enough?"

Intern: "Will I ever know enough?"

Resident: "Will I ever know enough?"

There really is more to learn than is humanly possible. You will do best to face this reality early on and settle for learning as much as you practically can. During the coming years, especially as you enter into clinical work, you will be able to fill many of the gaps in your knowledge.

Competition and Cooperation

For many entering students, medical school is an experience of second-class citizenship. For students accustomed to being unquestionably at the academic pinnacle, competing with classmates of similar abilities, some of whom have doctorates or master's degrees, can be unnerving. "Being the kind of conceited person I am, I have a high image of my intelligence and my ability to do things. But then the grades come out and I'm not at the top of the class where I should be." "I don't know if it's paranoia, but I feel that the other people are doing things and learning things that I'm not." "I've never considered myself conceited, but it was a real ego buster to suddenly not be effortlessly at the top of the heap. I had to deal with some Bs instead of straight As. I learned to forgive myself." "I've learned to lower my standards and to rationalize, 'Hey, this is med school; making Bs on tests is probably equivalent to As in college. You can't beat yourself up."

A few students, shaped by the premed syndrome, come to medical school with a "shark" mentality, a highly competitive mind-set, and sometimes undercut their classmates. "As an undergraduate I *never* had anyone sabotage an experiment or steal books, but it happened in medical school, starting with gross anatomy," one student lamented. "People stole dissecting atlases and mistreated other students' cadavers." "Our class was too competitive by nature. I found it very distasteful."

> Medical students probably remain competitive because they're used to getting As in college and don't know where they stand in med school. For example, during my second year a small group of students had the answers to histology slides and used them for exams without their classmates or instructors knowing.

DeWitt Baldwin, Steven Daugherty, Beverly Rowley, and Roy Schwartz at the American Medical Association (AMA) assessed cheating at 31 medical schools. They found that 5% of the students admitted they had cheated and 39% said they had witnessed their classmates cheating.[1] One student cautioned, "Cheating doesn't help because you do need to know the stuff. Even if you get by the course, you still have to know the material for the boards."

Two aspects of your medical education operate to your advantage. First, it's serial. As an entering student, you will learn from sophomores, juniors, seniors, and residents, recent survivors of the process you now experience. Their attitudes and advice can be invaluable. "More often than not, we teach each other." Second, it's collective. Everyone in your class will experience the same stress, status deprivation, academic pressure, and frustrations. "But many don't show it, and it can be very frustrating to think you're the only one having a difficult time." Your learning can be greatly enhanced by cooperating rather than competing. At some medical schools, each class annually revises, publishes, and disseminates for those who follow them a small booklet (*Sophomore Guide to Freshmen, Junior Guide to Sophomores,* etc.) that reviews each course and alerts students to basic problems and the best ways of handling them.

For some students, there is a reluctance to share intimate details of their initiation—whether through pride, forgetfulness, or a desire to pass on a good impression. "There is a real reluctance in medical school to call a spade a spade. People won't say that their experience was miserable because that implies that they weren't tough enough to take it." "In talking to friends," a third-year student reflected,

> I was amazed to find out that I wasn't the only one who went home and cried. But people don't let their guard down. Everyone tried to put up an "I know this" shield. But I've found that those who appear the most "I have it all together" actually have no clue when asked a question.

A graduating senior recalls,

It was socially unacceptable to complain to peers about the long hours, hard work, etc. When you did, they would ignore you or say, "Well, it's only going to get worse." I found this very strange, coming as it did from people who were undoubtedly experiencing the same feelings and stresses as me.

Cooperative classmates not only learn a great deal from one another but provide social support. An informal communication network benefits everyone:

Among my circle of friends, we share all our pains and stresses and support each other as much as possible. If someone has a death in the family or a personal problem, there's a lot of support—at least in my first year. I have been very unaware of the stigma of expressing weakness.

You may circulate information gleaned from old exams, lecture notes, and lab reports and share interesting experiences. To the consternation of some instructors, you may also divide up lab work, saving time without, it is to be hoped, curtailing learning. Although previous schooling has probably made you highly competitive, cooperation may become your best modus operandi: "If I find something significant on a histology test, I try to set up the one behind me by leaving the pointer on it."

Just studying with a classmate can resolve feelings of isolation and inadequacy. "I remember many times in anatomy when we taught each other. Late one Sunday night, a friend came to anatomy lab completely stressed that she didn't know the anatomy of the forearm. Two hours later, with some help, she knew a whole lot more and was less stressed out."

Status Deprivation

Almost every entering medical student feels keenly a sudden loss of status. "You were a college graduate last year, and here you are starting again as a lowly freshman." "We are the lowest of the low, and there are those who rub it in like salt into a wound." Knowing that you will eventually climb up the status ladder may comfort you. "Freshman medical students are lowest on the totem pole because they're just starting out and have four years to go. There isn't much further down to go, except maybe orderlies and freshman nurses.

But even the freshman nurses seem to have a lot more clinical training than we do."

Demeaning attitudes toward medical students impact their adjustment. "Since it takes a great deal of work to get in, and since all of us had to prove ourselves by competing with a lot of other capable, motivated people, we expected to be treated accordingly. All that goes out the window when you get into medical school." A female student married to a graduate student, contrasted her lot with her husband's:

> His situation is more of a peer relationship between the professors and graduate students. Classes consist of meeting at each other's houses, having dinner, and sitting around talking for a couple of hours. The faculty are his friends. It isn't a heavily structured situation like medical school. Here, we are not only treated like children, but also there is this rigid hierarchy and a somber authoritarian attitude that I just can't take seriously. Not only do they expect us to absorb all this technical information, but also they act like we don't know how to think, dress, or react in social situations. It's like we're coming in as blind slaves. It's just incredible!

To make matters worse, some first-year students perceive deliberate efforts by faculty members to humiliate them. "They treat us like dodos." "You get tired of being treated like a baby. On second thought, I wish we *were* treated as babies—don't you have to be nice to babies?"

A third-year student laments a "schizophrenic view of medical students":

> In my pediatric rotations, we were made to sit every other seat while taking the final exam. I was totally enraged, insulted, and dumbfounded that we were entrusted with human lives every day but could not, apparently, be trusted to be honest on an exam that only counted 10% of our final grade!

For women, the situation can be further aggravated when some male faculty members inject paternalism or sexual innuendo into the condescending way first-year medical students are treated. "When a woman asks a question or otherwise makes herself obvious, she is sometimes answered with an overly polite, condescending smile and tone as if we need to be coaxed!" Fortunately, many women find biased behavior the exception rather than the rule. In general, women are well respected and well regarded by faculty and students alike. And the majority of faculty and classmates apply pressure to those who fail to show proper respect. "One of my professors used a picture of a woman in seductive lingerie to illustrate an anatomy discussion—it didn't go over too well!"

There seems little doubt that faculty members in some schools emphasize status distinctions between themselves and first-year medical students quite deliberately. "In our clinical skills class, a female ophthalmologist said, 'I went through med school in 3 years; I've been doing this for 20 years; I know it all; you know nothing.' Right then and there I made mental note: Never ruin a teaching moment by humiliating people." Whether or not this treatment is useful in the process of creating doctors, entering students will likely experience it and will have to come to terms with it as it affects their work and self-image.

Fortunately, there are many exceptions to the model of the aloof, disinterested, or condescending, research-oriented instructor: "Some of them seem very interested and consider us intelligent. They have a job to do to get some information across and are generally happy they can do this." "Some of them really seem to want to help and explain things to you. I think they generally realize the student is yearning for knowledge." "There are many instances of basic science professors going out of their way to help students. And there are many students who are outright rude—snoring in class or leaving in the middle of the lecture."

Clinically Irrelevant Minutia

A common misconception is that "real medicine" will be taught from the beginning. Although this expectation prompts fears of harming patients through ignorance—"I don't know how I will treat a patient adequately without making a mistake"—its postponement is disappointing and frustrating. "Sometimes, I forget I'm in medical school—the class work seems pointed away from medicine." "I didn't think I'd be sitting behind a desk reading a book all the time, and I believed we'd use the stuff we learned more often. We just learn—period. We don't ever use it." And much of what is learned seems irrelevant to future practice. "It's trivia. Ninety-nine point nine percent of MDs, including profs, don't know the stuff they teach in med school unless they specialized in it."

The quality of the teaching is often disappointing. "I expected professors to be more interested in the students and to be more medically oriented." "I thought the professors here would be a long way from the caliber of my college professors—a lot smarter and more inspiring in the field they were in." "I find the faculty not as good as the majority of college instructors." "The professors need pedagogical training!" "I thought it would be more professionally carried out. Some things seem to be awfully Mickey Mouse." "The material is so disorganized you don't learn it; you just get used to it." "There seems to be no concept of matching teaching with the students' level or of progressing in an orderly manner." "I don't feel I'm getting that much out of classes. I really feel short changed."

Most professors are seen as generally well intentioned but aloof—"just doing their job; they see the year starting all over again, and they're going to go through the same thing they did last year." "You spend your college life taking all the hardest advanced courses. Then, you come to med school and learn all the medically related basic sciences—except they teach you in a remedial manner."

It's really true and unfathomable and preposterous that the basic science years of medical school are an academic let down. After my premed science courses and other college work, I imagined medical school as some kind of an exalted intellectual experience. Instead, it was in many ways absurd. You have to plow through masses of mostly trivial material, and the teaching is touch and go; it's tedious and frightening and annoying. Your anxiety and pressure are high. You feel weeks behind by the end of the second day. People fail tests. Don't worry too much: Simply work ridiculous amounts, take plenty of mental health breaks, and enjoy the camaraderie of your fellow drudges. At least, you all have lots in common.

Unfortunately for first-year students, the faculty members with whom they have the greatest contact are those least likely to be openly sympathetic to their specific concerns. "Basic scientists" are the PhDs who instruct first- and second-year students in medically oriented but nonclinical subjects such as gross anatomy, biochemistry, physiology, genetics, histology, microbiology, and neuroanatomy. They tend to be deeply imbedded in their own research and often regard teaching medical students (as opposed to specialized graduate students) as an intrusion on their time. Medical students readily recognize this attitude. "If you go up and ask a question, it's just a pain for them to explain something to you. They laugh and think you're stupid. One said to me, 'Have you considered another year of college?'"

At large institutions, students may be insulated from such attitudes of basic science faculty, seeing particular individuals only infrequently and having little direct contact with any of them. But in smaller schools, where faculty and students interact regularly, the relationship can be very strained. "In most courses, they compare their graduate students to medical students. They cater more to the graduate students and leave us out." "Some are quite helpful, but some feel that teaching us is a chore they have to put up with. They think every minute away from their research is a waste of time."

Graduate students hired to read and grade exams can exacerbate the problem:

> I got back a quiz where I'd obviously missed the question, and whoever graded the papers had written "UNBELIEVABLE" with a big exclamation point, and an X across the question, and that's all he put. I knew I'd missed the question, and if he'd just marked off the points I'd missed, okay. But he had to make a smart remark, and I think that's childish.

Because so much highly specialized information must be imparted to the students in a short time, the PhD-scientist-teachers often insist on memorization of details. "I thought I was done with regurgitation of extraneous material, but it's just beginning." Not only is it impossible for students to retain material learned this way, but it is difficult to relate it to clinical situations. "They give us a mass of material to memorize. If they would just point out things that are clinically applicable, we could better remember." "The information to be mastered is never 'prioritized.' Even though all the facts may be of equal importance to basic scientists, they are not equally important to a clinician."

Instructors vary in their efforts to translate valuable basic science material into clinically relevant contexts:

> For example, microbiologists organize bacteria by their physical characteristics, whereas clinicians organize them based upon which one is most likely to cause any given disease in any given situation. Hence, when you learn bacteriology in your second year, it doesn't seem clinically relevant. And once you hit the wards, the information as you learned it is not very helpful because it is in the wrong format.

Students are expected to assimilate a massive amount of scientific detail that seems irrelevant to clinical practice:

When PhDs lecture on an organism, they give you the size and shape—whereas we're more interested in knowing about the diseases it causes. We spent a whole lecture on a topic that has absolutely no bearing on patients. It's a purely scientific subject that the professor is doing his research on, so we had to learn it.

"Not even other professors in the same department know this stuff. It's crazy! They should make it optional, available to those who want it, like university courses."

It is frustrating when relevant information is not identified as such. "We performed an experiment in lab which, we later learned, can be used in diagnosing several different diseases; but we weren't told about any of them at the time. Knowing this would have given us a reference point and provided some meaning to the lab work."

Students' perceptions of the basic science faculty and their preoccupation with "irrelevant detail" are partially fostered by upper-division students, some clinical faculty members, and acquaintances who are practicing physicians. "The third year is when you get all the good stuff. That's what the upperclassmen tell us." "It's all part of the game," one clinician told some first-year students. "Learn it, regurgitate it, and forget about it, and you'll be all right." Another added, "Everything you learn the first two years is hogwash." "When I asked my [MD] freshman adviser what is relevant now, he said, 'None of it is.'"

They teach us about a lot of real weird diseases that are actually rare. I mentioned one to my Dad when I went home—the teacher had talked as if it were a common thing—but he said he'd been looking for a case ever since he got out of med school and had never seen one. We learn all these rare things, and then maybe spend 10 minutes on the common cold or sore throat.

"I couldn't wait to get to medical school and get down to the nitty-gritty—to the stuff that pertains to medicine. I haven't gotten there yet! It's been a semester and can't believe some of the stuff I've had to learn."

Although some of the "irrelevancy" argument is countered in schools where the first-year curriculum includes some clinical exposure and basic sciences are taught in connection with specific organ systems and functions, there is still a gulf between students and the ivory tower research scientists. "Basic scientists are just not rewarded for being good teachers. They are rewarded for their research." "Some of the basic science teachers have forgotten they're teaching med students; they're so engrossed in their own research they can't see why everyone isn't turned on by it." "They think they are brilliant and we're a bunch of stupid boobs who are eventually going to make more money than them."

Whatever their experience with professors, first-year students often reserve their highest praise for those few clinicians and faculty members who hold medical degrees. Most students are actively aware that this reflects their own tendency to identify with MDs and their preference for being taught by "someone who has done it, not just read about it." "They are really interested in getting up there and teaching you what medicine is about." "The MD is more interested in the student and better able to see what the problems of a medical student are, because he or she has been there."

> The medical faculty doesn't seem to have the specific knowledge that the science faculty has, but they give you more of an idea of what is going to be important to you and what you are going to get into when you start a practice. They may not be as well prepared, but they are a lot more interesting. And they like us better.

In an effort to improve the basic science curricula, most U.S. medical schools have implemented some of the educational strategies recommended in a report by the General Professional Education of the Physician (GPEP): decreasing lecture hours, introducing independent and small group learning experiences, integrating basic science and clinical education, using outpatient settings for clinical education, adding computer-based instruction, and promoting faculty mentorship and development programs.[2] Although reforms are limited by budgetary considerations, research priorities, and sturdy traditionalism, medical education is slowly becoming more user friendly.

Authoritarianism

One medical student compares medical training to military training. She says they both recruit young people full of leadership potential and essentially break their autonomous will through a rigorous hierarchy: "The first two years of medical training are boot camp, the last two, during which students are thrown onto the hospital wards, are definitely front-line duty."[3]

Ironically, the type of student attracted to medicine may be the least able to tolerate the indignities associated with being a medical student. Independent, self-motivated people often resent the authoritarianism that typifies medical school. Their reasons for choosing a medical career, as suggested by the following quotations, foreshadow adjustment problems: "I couldn't go into just any field where somebody would be telling me what to do." "I chose medicine for a career because I want to be my own boss." "I detest people ordering me around."

Students chafe under authoritarian instructors who insist on attendance and attention at lectures even by students who may already have done graduate work in the subject area. In some schools, attendance is only required at labs, and graduate students are exempt from taking courses in their areas of specialty. But in more authoritarian settings, an independent-minded student can suffer seemingly irrational requirements. "The first day of anatomy class the professor said, 'I feel that if you knew when to come to class and when not to, you'd be on the faculty and not a student, so we expect you to attend every class.'" "In biochemistry, one student who had taken the course in grad school was told he couldn't continue if he didn't attend lectures regularly. If the faculty has to be there, we have to be there too."

One of the professors in the histology department called me into his office and told me that because I hadn't been showing up to lab, the staff really wouldn't care to see me around next semester unless I change my ways. I thought I'd been better utilizing my time by studying the slides. I'd already taken histology in college and it was a much better course than his.

Faculty members at some schools seem to go to great lengths to extract attendance compliance from first-year students. One student was taken aback when the instructor "threatened to lower our exam grades by 15% if we missed two sessions of class. It was worse than being in kindergarten."

We had a micro test on Wednesday, and quite a few of the class had cut a lab on the previous day to study. On Monday morning the professor walked in and said he wanted our reports that day, though they weren't due until the following Wednesday. He did it for meanness, just to see if we'd done any work, and of course only a few of us had written up our notes.

Cadavers

As universally anticipated, first-year students dissect a cadaver in gross anatomy. It may be the students' first experience at handling a type of stress peculiar to the medical profession. For some students, the cadaver also represents the first direct experience with death. "I have never done anything like that before. It sort of made me sick to my stomach for a while." "It didn't really bother me at all until we got up to the face, and then it struck me for the second time that this is a human being I'm working on." "I didn't feel I would be upset by the cadaver, because it's pure science and all that. But it was a shock to walk in and see a body that you knew had once been living and you could have talked to before." "For the entire semester, you cannot get rid of the smell. It permeated everything: my clothes, my apartment, and me. Nothing helped." "We covered the face of our cadaver until the very end because it was too painful to look at." "It's a dehumanizing experience. There's a shock you can't express for fear of others around you." "I was most upset by other students who, in order to cope, had to give their cadavers cute names and treat them like old meat. It showed how much they were unwilling to confront reality."

Maureen Micek, a student at Dartmouth Medical School, kept a journal in which she included her reaction to gross anatomy. Here are a few excerpts:

Before, during, and after that first cut, I marveled at the level of trust the man who lived in this body—a complete stranger to me—must have had to offer his body up for dissection. Hadn't he been worried by the thought of his body falling into the hands of some gum- chewing, disrespectful premed who didn't give a damn about who he was, much less appreciate the enormous gift he had made?

. . . Dissection is a bittersweet experience. Part of it is gross. My stomach got a little queasy at the sight of fat cells oozing under my knife as I probed for the long thoracic nerve. But there was such fascination and pleasure from actually seeing the interior of the body. And I can think of no other way to gain this insight than to do the gross parts too.

. . . The face! Can you imagine dissecting a human face? The very idea is barbaric. Of course, any dissection of the human anatomy is a peculiar endeavor, but dissecting that part of the body which we so intimately connect with the person inside seems more than peculiar, it seems crude. . . .

It was hard going. I thought I had already been shocked enough times to be inured to this next step. I've sawed through skin and vertebrae to expose this man's spinal cord. I've dissected his penis and testicles, tugged at his pulmonary trunk, and palpated his intestines. All with care, all with respect. And I haven't had any nightmares about it. Instead of feeling guilt, I've felt gratitude. Instead of intimidation, I've felt excitement. But today I felt I was violating the man who gave us his body. I felt like I was stealing something precious that did not belong to me, rather than receiving a gift. A few hours after the lab ended, I told a friend it was as close to murder as I've ever come. I spend so much time reading people's faces, watching feelings cast over their eyes; if I've located the "person" anywhere in the body it's in the face especially the eyes. That's why it was so eerie watching the beam of a surgical lamp reflect off a human eyeball instead of seeing the gleam come from within. As I stared at a fully dissected cadaver later in the day, I felt primitive horror. No doubt dissecting the cadaver is a privilege, but there's a price one pays as well.[4]

Most students claim that the initial shock of working with a cadaver wears off quickly as they become immersed in learning the myriad details. "At my table people just dove in and cut; I myself was a 'cutter.' I thought people would be more hesitant, but I guess you're generally surrounded by Type-A gunner types and they all want to be the first." There is, however, an underlying current of medical machismo. To admit to being severely disturbed by the cadaver experience would be to display unphysicianlike emotion. "I often sense that we should have been born with the ability to be untouched by pain, suffering, and gore—and that admission to medical school should automatically grant one the ability to transcend normal human emotions."

Formal surveys and informal reports indicate that students are often deeply affected by dissection work. One author identified the psychic trauma evidenced by some as posttraumatic stress disorder.[5] Students' patterns of eating and sleeping were disturbed. Many reported nightmares linked to dissection and death. Some experienced upsetting visual images during the day. Anxiety and depression were also reported. "I didn't have any outward reservations about dissecting the cadavers," a fourth-year student recalled. "In fact, I was the one at our table who did the most dissecting. But I used to come to our lab with a feeling of dread. The experience is intense and draining and it's hard to deal with." "My grandmother passed away during anatomy. I had never had anyone close to me die. I will never forget touching her face at the funeral and realizing how odd it was, how so much like our cadaver. An eerie feeling remains with me today."

Fortunately, some schools are recognizing the impact of gross anatomy. Responding to a report from an anatomy TA that students were disturbed by their experiences, particularly with dissecting the hands, head, and neck, Stanford University students organized the Aid for the Impaired Medical Student (AIMS) Council. These students and faculty members sponsored a brown bag lunch. The son of a woman who had donated her body came to talk about her and alleviate their concerns. At the end of the anatomy course, the students held a memorial service, presided over by the university chaplin, that included student poetry.

Such programs provide a positive step in a field sometimes characterized by objectivity at the expense of humanity. In schools without a formal mechanism for discussing or evaluating the emotional impact of the cadaver experience, students are forced to objectify and intellectualize it on their own. Besides learning anatomy, students dissecting a cadaver actually undergo a socializing process, learning to behave and, to an extent, to feel as physicians rather than laypersons. As they participate in these rituals, students learn to detach themselves emotionally from the unpleasant experiences that are inescapable in clinical work. "For the first time in medical school, I have the sense I am being initiated into a priesthood," Perri Klass observed of her experiences with a human corpse: "This is something that normal people never do."[6] "But," another trainee pointed out, "It's the first thing they ask of med students."

Emotional Crisis

The sudden overwhelming occurrence of status loss, new environments, changed relationships, heavy academic pressures, and confrontations with death can unsettle even a relatively placid personality. After an initial period of shock and depression, most students regain their perspective. But some struggle continuously through all four years. "I consider dropping out every Monday morning," a fourth-year student said, "but I have only four months left to do it."

Time constraints are a recurrent problem for all students. "Even though I more or less knew the curriculum, I didn't expect such a small amount of time for personal things," one said. "There's more of everything than I expected."

"Finding a balance between school and life has been a goal since day one," said a third-year student. "I'm not there yet."

Many students fail to adjust satisfactorily because they have no ready avenue for sharing and thus relieving their frustrations and anxieties. And some students, unprepared intellectually and emotionally for the realities of medical school, simply opt out. Twenty to 30% of the students seek assistance from staff psychiatrists, and many others may get professional attention outside the school environment. "Due to my difficulty in dealing with my father's death, I did seek out help. We dealt with the grief and then all these other emotions—fear, anxiety, roommate problems—came spilling out. It really helped me to talk with a third party." There are those, however, who may need help but hesitate to ask for it; they are reluctant to reveal feelings of personal inadequacy for fear that disclosure may become part of their official record and jeopardize an already tenuous status. "There is a fear that you will be asked to leave once they discover how you really feel."

A study of 286 students at Duke University School of Medicine found decreases in all of 10 aspects of physical and emotional health during the first year of medical training. The most significant change was an increase in depression.[7] At Louisiana State University School of Medicine, another study also found impaired emotional well-being among first-year medical students. Students experienced a loss of control, self-esteem, and uplifts and decreases in positive moods: joy, contentment, vigor, and affection. They also felt hassled, depressed, and sometimes hostile.[8] Robert Pasnau, a psychiatrist who directs a counseling program for medical students notes that (a) medical trainees are as mentally healthy as the general population, and (b) the most common problem is "adjustment disorder with depressed mood."[9]

Given these facts, it is surprising that relatively few medical schools offer preventive programs to help students deal with the psychosocial impact of their experience, for example, programs of primary prevention such as activities sponsored by the Student Well-being Committee at the University of California, Los Angeles[10] and at the Mt. Sinai School of Medicine.[11] "With the second suicide in two years here, I hope this is changing. I think they are learning that students need support and they are encouraging us to use counseling services."

Generally, the formal emphasis is on developing a "scientific attitude," and although faculty specialists are available when all else fails, many students feel they are left to deal as best they can with their feelings. "Often, I sense that there is no official recognition that feelings even exist—as if they are nonentities—or that only a woman like me could care about such unscientific concerns."

> Really, there's no one at the medical center to talk to. You feel as though it will be fed back to the administration and indicate you are having difficulty handling the material. And, possibly, in the long run, they might boot you if something happened or make you repeat a course. It could be something that could be used against you.

Most students experience the same feelings, and a supportive network of peers can ease the pressure. "My friends and I constantly remind each other how smart we are. At least, it makes us laugh at our insecurities." The Duke University study previously cited found that social support was a key factor among medical students whose health and life attitude remained positive during the first year. Adequate sleep and regular physical exercise were also significant health determinants.[12] "In my class we had numerous people run the LA marathon, compete in triathalons. It's those people who are most organized and do better."

Some schools offer significant social support at times of crises.

> Fortunately, the school was very understanding when there was a death in my family. I missed a week of classes but they faxed me lecture notes upon request. My professors and the Student Affairs Office called my parent's home to see how I was. Classmates sent flowers. When I came back, my anatomy professor put me in a tutorial group for those students who had had difficulty with the midterm (I had not, but it was to help me catch up). All of this happened when we were doing the face. I honestly told my professor that I didn't know if I could cope with being in lab. He told me to take my time and I didn't need to go. I ended up going and my partners were excellent in reviewing the material.

Lest this picture of medical school as a potential thief of health and humanity seem too pessimistic, keep in mind that not all is gloomy. By capturing the feel of student frustrations, I hope to spare you later disillusionment, not create anticipatory anxieties. The good news is that all but a few make it to graduation, some of whom, like this graduating senior, are exhilarated by the training experience:

I agree it was a tough time—socially, intellectually, and emotionally—but, in retrospect, it was also the best time of my life. I've acquired some of my best friends, shared some incredible times, and developed intellectually and emotionally at an accelerated rate. Fortunately, our medical school has made an attempt to provide support for us during trying times; the associate deans have always stressed that their doors are open, and the psychiatrists have offered free group sessions and/or individual counseling. Even if I were to quit medical school today, five months before graduation, I would not regret the experience.

Insights: Are Emotions Bad?
Bernard Virshup, MD

One of the elements that can sear humanity out of medical students is the general medical ambiance of unemotionality. Doctors like to invoke the concept of "professional distance," rationalizing that this helps them stay uninvolved and therefore better able to handle the stresses of medicine. If you have feelings about things, better not show it; even better, don't have feelings. This implies that it is impossible for physicians to learn to handle emotional stress. As a result, they lose authenticity, are unable to deal with feelings, and have difficulty relating to ordinary people who have lots of feelings.

Holding feelings in check for a lifetime is destructive. You must practice expressing them, if possible to those who will be supportive, but even to those who will not. Many of the feelings you will have in the course of your career will be painful. Shame, self-doubt, humiliation, embarrassment, and many other feelings will come up. What are you to do with them? You won't, of course, share them with patients; you won't share them with people who might criticize you for having them. It is, however, absolutely necessary that you acknowledge these feelings to yourself and accept yourself for having them.

The first week of medical school, you are introduced to your cadaver, which you skin. Most medical students walk into the anatomy lab filled with uncomfortable feelings—some expressing themselves in physical symptoms like nausea. Most try not to show these feelings. With bland expressions and clenched teeth, they pretend they're just fine. Start by reassuring yourself that the feelings you have when you see your cadaver are normal, and you are normal for having them; that you would not be human if you didn't have such feelings; that others are also having them; and that you can and will live to tolerate them. Indeed, you will come to be grateful that you can and do have these feelings.

What you must do is be able to talk to someone about these feelings, people who will understand them and accept you and perhaps even be willing to share their own feelings. Who better than the other medical students at your dissection table?

Share those feelings. Let your group know what is going on with you. It will almost certainly evoke similar feelings in the others, who will be grateful that you broke the ice.

This doesn't mean that you should burden everyone all the time with all your feelings. But you should regularly unburden yourself to at least a select few. Not all your feelings will be bad. There are many wonderful feelings, some approaching epiphany. Share these feelings, too.

To share your feelings, you have to know what they are. One good way to stay in touch with your feelings is to query yourself regularly, "How do I feel about this?" Every morning, before rushing off to school, take a moment to ask yourself, "How do I feel this morning?"

Have a wide range of apparel to reflect your feelings. Wear clothes that shout your feelings, good or bad. If you are a man, and if your school makes you wear ties, have a wide range of them, so that every morning you can reflect for a moment, "Which do I feel like today?"

Drawings can reflect feelings. Take a few minutes every day to create a quick picture of your mood. Pick your colors, make your strokes to reflect how you feel. You don't have to be an artist to do this—what you draw is less important than how you draw it. Label each drawing with the event about which you are having feelings and save the drawings. They will form a record for you of your trip through medical school.

All the arts can serve this function. Music is the ultimate way to tap into and express your feelings. Poetry, and especially a poetry group, is effective for many; dance is effective for others. All these can reflect feelings, even feelings you may not know you have.

Be aware of your body, and whether it is a heavy burden or is moving with a light step. Move the way you feel.

Several times a day, check into yourself, and say to someone, "I feel . . . ," and fill in the blank.

Notes

1. Baldwin, DeWitt, Steven R. Daugherty, Beverly D. Rowley, and M. Roy Schwartz. 1996, March. "Cheating in Medical School: A Survey of Second-Year Students at 31 Schools." *Academic Medicine,* 71(3):267-273, p. 4.

2. Jonas, H. S., S. I. Etzel, and B. Barzansky. 1989. "Undergraduate Medical Education. Section 1: Medical Education." *Journal of the American Medical Association,* 262(8):1011-1019, p. 1018.

3. DasGupta, Sayantani. 1996, November. "A Bitter Bullet." *The New Physician,* pp. 11-12, p. 11.

4. Micek, Maureen. 1987, September. "Invasion." *The New Physician,* pp. 15-16, p. 15.

5. Finkelstein, Peter. 1986. "Studies in the Anatomy Laboratory: A Portrait of Individual and Collective Defense." In Robert H. Coombs, D. Scott May, and Gary W. Small, eds. *Inside Doctoring: Stages and Outcomes in the Professional Development of Physicians* (pp. 22-42). New York: Praeger.

6. Klass, Perri. 1987. *A Not Entirely Benign Procedure.* New York: NAL/Signet.

7. Parkerson, George R., Jr., W. E. Broadhead, and Chiu-Kit J. Tse. 1990. "The Health Status and Life Satisfaction of First-Year Medical Students." *Academic Medicine,* 65(9):586-587.

8. Wolf, T. M., T. K. Von Almen, J. M. Faucett, H. M. Randall, and F. A. Franklin. 1991. "Psychosocial Changes During the First Year of Medical School." *Medical Education,* 25:174-181.

9. Lowes, Robert. 1995, November. "Edge of Darkness." *The New Physician,* pp. 18-27, p. 19.

10. Coombs, Robert H., and Bernard Virshup. 1994. "Enhancing the Psychological Health of Medical Students: The Student Well-Being Committee." *Medical Education* [Special issue on medical student well-being], 28:47-54.

11. Lowes, *op. cit.*

12. Parkerson, Broadhead, and Tse, *op. cit.*

CHAPTER 3

Student Diversity
Who Are All These People?

We have a large melting pot in our class—people of every race, color, and creed imaginable. Sometimes, people don't understand each other and are offended, but we get exposure to a large number of people that will help to prepare for different kinds of patients.

—31-year-old medical student

Born Loser

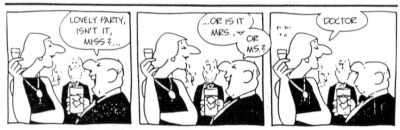

Medical school used to be the exclusive domain of white males—mostly young, single, and affluent, with undergraduate degrees in biology or another branch of science. Times have changed. Today's beginning medical student may be a single Latina parent, an African American liberal arts graduate, a grandmother, a disabled Asian American, a lesbian, or an engineer with several years of work experience. "I sometimes feel like a token white girl," said a student at a highly diversified medical school.

Ethnic and religious ties, socially reinforcing for some students, also accentuate their visibility to classmates. "The Jewish students tend to stick together," one observed. "The minority students sit apart from the main class." "At our school, the African American students keep to themselves." "There are 10 of us Chicanos in the class; I'm the oldest, and we have get-togethers every other week. We really enjoy the interaction."

Another prominent division you will likely observe is married versus unmarried. "It's a natural clique," one student said. Married students tend to spend leisure time with spouses and families more than with their classmates and "to hang out with other married students." "They have their own parties and stuff." "A friend of mine brought his wife over from Iran, and now there's one less person to get pizza with. Wedding bells are breaking up that old gang of mine."

Some medical schools located in heterogeneous cities pride themselves on their diverse student body. "On the first day of class," one student reported,

we were asked, "Raise your hand if you were born in a different country." About half of us did. People have come from all over the world. They're not foreigners, but they're Americans now. When you start talking to them and hear their stories, you realize they are really quite unique. Since I, too, came from another country, I felt for the first time, "Maybe I really am where I belong." Even though we might come from different parts of the world, we're together now.

You will be spending four intense years with diverse individuals in your medical school class and the challenging residency years with others like them. Eschew the cutthroat mentality of a shortsighted few; you will dissect your first cadaver with these people, lose countless hours of sleep studying with them, celebrate passing exams with them, and survive clinical rounds with them. They are likely to be your primary source of support, and you theirs; who else will possibly understand what you're going through, let alone not get weary of talking about it? But even as you share common struggles, you'll find that you and some of your classmates confront unique challenges.

The other chapters focus on experiences common to most, if not all, medical students. But by way of introducing you to your medical school companions, this chapter takes a look at the medical school experience through the eyes of a few subgroups: women, racial and ethnic minority students, students with disabilities, gay and lesbian students, and older students.

Women Students

The first woman physician in the United States, Dr. Elizabeth Blackwell, was initially refused admission to medical schools, so she studied privately until 1847, when she finally entered Geneva Medical School in New York. After graduation, she studied in London. When she returned home, she was denied all hospital or clinic positions she applied for. Undeterred, she and her sister opened a medical dispensary and staffed it entirely with women. "It is hard with no support but a high purpose," she said, "to live against every species of social opposition."[1] One physician tells of a gift that, for her, summarizes the situation of a woman in medicine in the 1960s. It was the gift her grandmother gave her for graduating from medical school, a silver tea set.

> No doubt she confused my future life with the life of the doctors' wives she had known: supported by servants, having friends in for tea and serving in the socially graceful Southern style. I've often thought of that tea set when in the midst of some operating room disaster, bathed in blood and sweating to keep a difficult patient alive and defended from the surgeon's assault. My grandmother must have felt it was acceptable for a woman to get a M.D. degree but must have felt subconsciously that a woman doctor should live the gracious life of the doctor's *wife,* not the doctor's *life,* up all night saving a patient's life, a life with no time for afternoon tea or pleasant social chatting. This incongruity between the social side of life—especially meeting family responsibilities—and professional life—what doctors do each day—continues for me and most other women physicians to the present time.[2]

With affirmative action, the number of women physicians increased dramatically in the past two decades, according to the American Medical Association's (AMA) statistics. Contributing to this acceleration were 1970 class action complaints against every medical school in the country filed by the Women's Equity Action League.[3] Although the total number of physicians went from 334,028 in 1970 to 653,062 in 1992—not quite doubling in 22 years—figures for women physicians for the same period increased nearly fivefold from 25,401 to 118,519.[4]

In 1994, first-year women students at Yale School of Medicine outnumbered men for the first time—at 56% of the entering class. This phenomenon was noted at 17 other schools among the 126 medical schools in the nation. Overall, women recently have made up about 42% of applicants and students admitted to medical schools for the past three years.[5] By the year 2010, 30% of all doctors are projected to be female, most of them practicing family medicine.[6] "I know more and more female surgeons and subspecialists," a resident observed:

One night around 2 a.m. I went to the Emergency Department [ED] to do a neurology consult. I was quite amused to recognize that every doc in the room, from the ED attending to the medical students; and all of us subspecialty residents happened to be women. Better yet, no one else would have noticed how unusual that was until I pointed it out.

Changing expectations about women's roles also contributed to the influx of women in medicine. Speaking at a college commencement, the Supreme Court Justice Sandra Day O'Connor recalled that after her 1952 graduation from Stanford Law School her only job offer from the private sector was as a legal secretary. That same year, the presidential candidate Adlai Stevenson encouraged the female student body at Smith College to be proud of their accomplishments and to use their education to improve the world by influencing their husbands and sons to succeed. "Isn't it wonderful that that address will never again be given in the United States?" exclaimed Justice O'Connor. "Today, young women are expected to have, and do have, a direct influence on public affairs. There are more women in public office, in state and national legislative positions, than ever before and there are more women candidates for public office at all levels of government than ever before in our history."[7]

O'Connor told the 2,428 graduates, 1,137 of whom were women, "As students today, your challenges will not come so much in breaking new paths as your mothers, grandmothers, and I've done, but in deciding which of the many paths now open you should choose from. As far as I'm concerned, it is worth every bit of the extra effort I've put into it to have a family as well as a career. . . . As for women today, the tide is running in your favor; the wind is at your back."[8]

Nevertheless, as a woman medical student you may still experience significant gender-related struggles. A University of Texas study shows that male and female medical students enter medical school with comparable mental health and similar levels of life satisfaction. Beginning the first year of medical school, however, women report more depression, more anxiety, and less satisfaction with their lives.[9]

Gender-related struggles typically occur in one of four ways. First, women encounter subtle and overt forms of sexism, harassment, and discrimination from male colleagues, hospital staff, and patients. Second, women experience the basic stresses of medical school and medical practice differently from men. Third, many women bear responsibilities of home and family that their male counterparts do not. And fourth, in academia women physicians tend to be promoted less often than men.

Sexism, officially disapproved, still exists. One third of the women at a large midwestern university said they had experienced discrimination in medical school and nearly two thirds (64%) observed gender discrimination toward classmates, particularly during their clinical rotations. In addition, one third of the women were sexually harassed by someone in a position of authority, and nearly half by a fellow student.[10] "Women don't belong in medicine, much less in surgery," a female surgery resident was told by an attending surgeon. "All women physicians are hysterical."[11] A prominent neurosurgeon, Frances Conley, fought back in 1991, attracting national attention by resigning from the faculty of Stanford University School of Medicine when a man she believed devalued women was named department chair. He had, she said, subjected her for 25 years to sexist remarks and unwarranted sexual advances.[12]

Despite the 50-50 ratio of men to women in one medical student class, a student notes that gender distinction "affects every single thing you can think of": "The very first day one of the physicians was lecturing on the breast and him saying, 'Its smooth, lovely contour,' stuff like that. Some of the more militant women in the class—or braver maybe—said, 'Excuse me, do you mind?'"

In an article titled "Tales out of Medical School," Adrianne Fugh-Berman reports that an overwhelmingly white, male, and conservative faculty at her medical school,

> built disrespect for women into its curriculum. The prevailing attitude towards women was demonstrated on the first day of classes by my anatomy instructor, who remarked that our elderly cadaver "must have been a playboy bunny" before instructing us to cut off her large breasts and toss them into a 30 gallon trash can marked "cadaver waste." Barely hours into our training, we were already being taught that there was nothing to learn from examining breasts, despite that one out of nine women develop breast cancer. An appalling waste of an educational opportunity.[13]

One student noted this blatant sexism:

> I think if I had been prettier I would have had more problems. On ortho surgery I felt like a visiting mascot for these big strong guys. They would

say sexist things about their girlfriends or who they were sleeping with. They would either forget I was there or consider me one of the gang and not think I would be bothered by it.

A female resident commented, "It amazes me that in educated professional circles it's acceptable to make jokes at the expense of women. And yet the analogous jokes about racial minorities are strictly taboo. And when we object, they accuse us of being hysterical.[14]

Medical students are conditioned to be tough, macho, and silent in the face of challenges and to never admit that they "don't have what it takes" to make it in medical school. When women protest sexist behaviors, they may be called "hysterical," "whining," "bitch," "dragon lady"—words never used to describe men.

One day I was called into the chairman's office and told I was "bitchy, aggressive and difficult to get along with." I was then scheduled for the department's equivalent of Siberia, the nearby eye institute. By this time, I had changed enough to realize that to be called "bitchy, aggressive and difficult to get along with" meant I had grown from a painfully shy, quiet woman. I now had the same skills as a strong man, who would be described as "aggressive, strong and effective"—because these traits are seen as good in men, but bad in women.

When the medical student Shelby Rush campaigned for a leadership position in AMSA, her ability to perform was questioned because she was pregnant. She notes,

Women are questioned and remain suspect because of their child-bearing capacity. Yet I have never heard of a man being asked his family plans during a job interview. It is important to be aware of our prejudices and learn about all types of discrimination—not to pretend they don't exist. It happened to me. It happened within AMSA.[15]

"Women in research tell of being denied promotions and tenure because of leave time they use to have a baby," Rush notes. She continues,

Female residents are forced to take double call while pregnant to make up for maternity leave later. Men who miss time because of illness—a broken leg or hepatitis for example—do not face these problems. . . .

Pregnancy and parenthood are not diseases, but they do deserve the same allowances and work considerations as unplanned illnesses.[16]

Edith Gross examined differences in perceived sources of stress among male and female physicians and found that both reported time demands were their biggest stressor.[17] Women especially felt completely bereft of personal time. In addition to the ordinary stresses of medicine, women struggle with the sense that they must represent their gender. They feel the need not only to succeed but to outdo their male colleagues, all the while showing no sign of mental fatigue.

In the same study, male physicians reported significantly more strain due to relationships with patients than did female physicians—51.5% compared to 17.9%. When women physicians found patient relations a source of stress, it was because they felt emotionally drained by the demands of sick patients or patients' parents. In contrast, male physicians complained about "difficult," "demanding," "inconsiderate," or "bitchy" patients, those who showed "a lack of appreciation" or "lack of trust." Gross explains:

> The fact that male physicians are more likely to be vexed by the doctor-patient relationship than female physicians is related not only to their status as physicians, but also to their status as men in a sex-stratified society. The role of the doctor traditionally has been one of high prestige and authority, as has the role of the male in society generally. Thus as physicians and as males, they expect to be granted a degree of deference and power. Studies show that male students are more likely than female to hold the so-called traditional belief in physician authority.[18]

Some nurses treat women physicians with less deference and respect than men, regardless of their professional training and role. Nurses typically help male doctors and clean up after themselves but they may not for women. "I have found in my own training," said Perri Klass, a pediatrician, "that nurses generally expect me to clean up after myself . . . to do a fair amount of my own secretarial work," and to act humbly, "not to take a too high and mighty tone."[19]

Patients sometimes slight women doctors by assuming they are nurses or discounting their work. Dr. Barbara Ross-Lee, dean of the Ohio University College of Osteopathic Medicine, had a patient refuse her diagnosis until it was confirmed by a male physician, one of her students.[20]

Women's traditionally lower status may make it easier for them to interact with patients whose egalitarian views of physicians can threaten male doctors. This Chinese American woman medical student understands the need for flexibility: "I don't want to be a stickler for tradition," she noted. "Sometimes, being too bent on keeping the status quo is not good. The world is changing around you and if your mind is set—'I was trained to be this way'—and you refuse to adjust, it might not be the best way to help your patient."

Financing medical education is another area of disproportionate stress for women. According to Clark, "Women seemed to be under greater financial pressure in medical school, entering medical school with more debt and 79% reporting financial trouble compared to 58% of the men."[21]

Women may not have the option to adopt the work-first orientation of their male counterparts because of family and household responsibilities. Men generally expect that a wife will be the homemaker and child rearer, but women rarely make such assumptions about their husbands. Most female physicians' husbands are employed (92.6%). Less than half of male physician's wives are employed (45%).[22] Unless they remain single and childless, women must merge career development and family obligations, with the accompanying role conflict and increased psychological stress. As Dr. Bernadine Healy, who directed the National Institutes of Health remarks, "Women are still the primary nurturing force within the family."[23]

A married woman student commented that during an evening study session a married male colleague called his wife, a schoolteacher, and asked her to bring him a pizza. She bundled their child into the car, got the pizza, and delivered it to the group. The woman student was amazed, for her husband was at home, displeased that she wasn't there to cook for him.

Working two jobs is a strain on anyone; but the intense time and energy demands of a physician make "the second shift" on the home front particularly burdensome for women doctors. The powerful societal expectation that women will care for the home regardless of any other commitment profoundly impacts the way women physicians conduct their medical careers and the rewards they receive for their efforts.

A mother of a young child compromised:

In anesthesia we had a case that required reading five articles before surgery in the morning. I made up my mind that I could spend more time with my family if I only did three of them. I didn't meet their standard and was not considered chief resident material. On the other hand, I thought, "I don't need that. I can still be a good anesthesiologist without being the chief. I'm going to have a healthy baby and marriage."

Many women in medicine cope with the career-family dilemma by selecting a specialty compatible with family life. Women are three times more likely than male physicians to be pediatricians and half as likely to be surgeons. Women physicians enter academic medicine in greater percentages than their male counterparts, but in U.S. medical schools they still represent only 20% of full-time faculty.[24]

As practicing physicians, are women paid the same for equal work? The pediatrician Marilyn Gaston, director of the U.S. Bureau of Primary Health Care, reports having been paid less than her male counterparts. When she objected, she was told that she had a husband and that the men had families to support.[25] Lawrence Baker points out that whereas in the early 1980s female physicians earned about 13% less per hour than men, at the time of his study men and women beginning their medical careers earned the same amount when factors such as hours worked weekly and differences in specialty and practice settings were considered. Baker found that, on the average, men put in more work time and were more likely to specialize in fields like cardiology with higher pay. But pay inequity existed for older physicians. Even when type of practice and hours worked are considered, men with 10 or more years of experience earned 17% more per hour than their female counterparts.[26]

Women in academic medicine are promoted more slowly than men according to an Association of American Medical Colleges (AAMC) survey of men and women who had been on a medical school faculty for an average of 11 years. Eighty-three percent of men compared to only 59% of women had achieved associate or full professor rank. This distinction could not be explained by productivity or differential attribution.[27]

Do women bring unique strengths to the practice of medicine? Most studies find more similarities than differences in the ways men and women approach medical practice. As medical students they perform similarly in almost all areas. Since women may be more inclined to seek female physicians to deliver their children and take care of their health, however, women physicians may be highly marketable in today's world. Plus, there is anecdotal evidence that women seek female physicians because of their greater compassion and understanding.[28] One study shows that women physicians spend more time with patients—17 minutes compared to men's 13 minutes. Another study, at Johns Hopkins University, showed that patients talk to women physicians 40% more than they do men doctors.[29] The Council on Graduate Medical Education (COGME) notes that many female physicians' practice styles can result in better communication with patients and increased overall patient satisfaction.[30]

According to the COGME, women are more likely than men to enter medical education for altruistic reasons rather than financial ones.[31] Students at a southwestern state medical school responded to a 57-item questionnaire to assess their opinions and attitudes about providing care to medically underserved populations. Women were consistently more favorably inclined toward providing these basic services.[32] Earlier findings also show that female physicians generally are more liberal, egalitarian, and sensitive than male physicians and that after controlling for the age of a physician, gender accounts for more variability in attitudes than medical specialty.[33]

Racial and Ethnic Minorities

Racial and ethnic minority students made up 12.2% of all medical students in 1996—a record high but still far short of the original goal of 3,000 underrepresented minorities by the turn of the century set by the AAMC so that all patients can be served by physicians who understand them and their culture. Reaching this goal may be difficult in light of recent political attacks on affirmative action policies. The number of blacks, Latinos, and Native Americans applying to the University of California (UC) medical schools dropped 22% in the year following a decision by the UC regents forbidding consideration of race or ethnicity in UC admissions, along with passage of Proposition 209, which banned race and gender preferences in the California schools. "I'm not sure we're declaring surrender," said Herbert Nickens, the AAMC vice president in charge of community and minority programs, "but it's looking more and more difficult. No one who is committed to this issue is going to give up."[35]

It is not true that to assemble an ethnically diverse student body a medical school must accept minority students who do not meet minimum academic standards. At the University of California, for example, more than 95% of all students admitted are chosen from the top 12.5% of the state's high school graduates, regardless of race or ethnicity. Only 5% are admitted by exception. Affirmative action proponents believe that a diverse undergraduate and medical school student body is important because (a) graduates serve a more heterogenous patient population, and (b) they make college more socially and academically rigorous. "You learn more from those who do not think as you do, from those who have had very different life experiences," said Jean H. Fetter, a former dean of undergraduate admission at Stanford. "Students in homogenous classes do not offer each other much potential for learning."[36]

Complaints about affirmative action fall into two categories: first, a perception that, following admission, affirmative action students have access to special programs. In the competitive environment of medicine, any perceived perk or advantage to one group is resented by another. The privileged who enjoyed years of superior educational opportunities may perceive as unfair a short-term tutoring program for economically and educationally deprived students:

> At my med school, they offer a summer course to entering minority students that teaches them how to study and gives them basic information about the first few weeks of school. By the time school starts, they're way ahead of the game! One friend told me he received information based solely on his Hispanic surname. Medical school in general was stressful and having to deal with people who were primed with advance information made me feel like I didn't know anything. I learned quickly to stay away from them to maintain my sanity!

Neither did minority students like this special attention: "I had always excelled and was confident," a Latina remarked, "but this gave me the feeling that automatically there was something inherently lacking in me." "It labeled us as educationally handicapped," another complained, "it stereotyped us."

Other concerns are about admission preferences. An unsuccessful applicant expressed his bitterness this way:

> I'm just an average Anglo-Saxon Protestant male, and that was not in vogue at the time I was applying. If two students are equally qualified to enter medical school, and it is the policy of the medical school to accept minority students in an effort to bring racial minority doctors up to their percentage in the population, I'd step aside and say, "Fine; I'm for that any time." But when you drop qualifications for any particular religious or racial group, then you're diluting the quality of medical education and, ultimately, the quality of medical care.

In reaction to this view, an African American applicant points out,

If it's hard for white men and women to get in, then it's three times as hard for us. Everybody is using this reverse discrimination argument: "A minority got your seat." But look at it. Of all the medical schools in the nation, only a small percentage of the seats are filled by minorities. It isn't right!

Indeed, it does seem stingy of the majority to covet those few spots.[37] But covet they do. "The reverse discrimination theme has built momentum and closed a lot of doors to us," said an unsuccessful black woman applicant.

Some Asian American students maintain they are discriminated against because of their success. "To get into medical school is harder if you are Asian," one said. "The expectations are much higher from the administration and from parents." An Asian American woman agreed. "It's harder for an Asian man to get into med school than a white man because there are so many well-qualified Asian males and admissions committees don't want half the class to be Asian."

Ironically, minority students who have not benefited from affirmative action programs often find themselves targets of resentment. "They are shocked when I tell them that I have a 3.5 GPA and received 14s and 15s on the MCAT (Medical College Admission Test)," one reported. Speaking of minority students in her class, a black woman commented,

The idea is still pervasive that blacks aren't as capable in medical school as whites. White students assume we're getting extra tutoring, which we aren't. Some of us are getting As in courses like anatomy and histology, and the white students don't expect this. They thought we'd remain at the bottom. Even if they didn't have the grades coming in, the black and Chicano students here still achieve as well as the white students.

How capable are minority students? The performances of 42 underrepresented minorities and 368 other students who graduated from the University of Arizona College of Medicine between 1987 and 1991 were compared. Although the students from underrepresented minorities entered medical school with significant educational disadvantages and continued to score lower than the other students on paper-and-pencil tests, their clinical performances on the Objective Structured Clinical Examination (OSCE) and family practice clerkship were nearly equivalent to those of the other students.[38]

Sometimes, their success comes from working harder than other students, as this black woman graduate student preparing to reapply to medical school explained:

> I graduated from an inner-city high school with a 3.9. So I came to the university thinking I was doing great. What I didn't know was that my 3.9 was equivalent to about a 2.9 in other schools. So I came with a tremendous disadvantage in basic academic preparation. I not only had to keep up with what the professor was doing in class, I had to go back and make up what I had missed in high school. And while I was doing that, students who didn't have makeup work were in the library doing extra things. My GPA now reflects that disadvantage. Also, I've always had to work 30 hours or more a week. You have to be very strong to handle all the pressure.

Some students are uncertain whether affirmative action decisions are based on race or deprivation—and are more comfortable with the idea of the latter. An Asian student notes, "Affirmative action nowadays might be better defined in terms of socioeconomic status. The idea is to give people who are disadvantaged a possibility of working toward some professional goal. Just because you're Hispanic doesn't mean you were extremely poor and never had opportunities."

According to one study, parents' income significantly relates to medical students' performance on the MCAT and the U.S. Medical Licensing Examination (USMLE) regardless of gender or racial or ethnic status. Students with more parental resources, regardless of racial or ethnic group, are better able to cope with unexpected expenses and buy supplemental educational materials. Also, poorer students are more likely to hold outside employment or use some of their financial aid to augment family incomes.[39]

Students in the majority culture sometimes suspect minority students of exaggerating or whining in an undoctorlike way when they report incidents of discrimination. Most minority students, however, do experience belittling and stereotyping from early on. A Latina student recalls:

> At the end of my freshman year in high school, I went in to set up my schedule for the next three years. I wanted college prep courses. There was no question that I was going to be a doctor. My counselor looked at me and said, "You're nothing but a dumb Mexican and that's all you're ever going to be. The Mexicans around here get home economics for the

girls and if you're a boy you get auto body, and that's what you're going to get." I looked at him and said, "Excuse me, did you just say what I thought you said? "Yup, that's what I said." I walked out of the office, down the hall, and called my Mom at work. "Mom, Mr. —— just called me a dumb Mexican and said that's all I'd ever be." CLICK! I went out in front and waited. Ten minutes later my Mom pulled up going about 50 mph. She didn't even close the car door she was so angry. I did get the courses I wanted and took college prep classes at a local junior college at night when I was a sophomore and eventually graduated from high school as a junior.

Discrimination often occurs unintentionally, as in this Chicano medical student's experience:

Where I grew up, it's a two-class system—rich whites and poor Hispanic farmworkers. Regardless of my achievements in college, people still see me as the latter. During my surgery internship at a local hospital, one of the surgeons explained to a staff member that we were going to do a procedure using the endoscope and asked him to show me how to work with it before we actually got started. The staff person started showing me how to clean the endoscope and sweep the floor. I was wearing scrubs, yet he assumed that I was going to clean the equipment and sweep the floors!

Unfortunately, his experience is not unique. This fourth-year resident had a similar experience:

I remember coming out of the surgery suite dressed in scrubs and was clearly part of the team. Someone—for reasons I don't know—mistook me for housekeeping and demanded that I pick up some dirty laundry. It was the ultimate embarrassment. Here I was trying to talk to the residents and attendings and this person is shouting at me to pick up some laundry!

Prejudice and discrimination add to already stressful lives. "I came to California because I wanted to get away from racial discrimination in the South," said a black student. "There discrimination is rednecked, in jeans and cowboy hats. Here it comes in business suits and doctor's whites—very much in disguise."

Majority medical students may find themselves in an embarrassing situation when they are unaware of their own prejudices and fail to keep them out of the examination rooms. A top administrator of a major medical school broke her arm and was being treated by an Anglo resident. He told her to "hold her arm up like she'd hold a beer can on a Saturday night." The black female administrator exploded, "What are you talking about? You think I'm a welfare mother?" The physician shrugged, "Well, aren't you?" Wrong. She was the associate dean. Oops!

Experiences like these remind many minority students they are perceived first as members of a minority and second as medical students. And they constantly deal with stereotypes. The more stoic minority students may be used to prejudicial treatment and often have quiet strategies for combating its effects:

> You never want to come off as being "that silly black student" making jokes all the time and never acting seriously. Even though you may be the smartest, most serious student in the class and do your work to a high standard, they won't remember that. They'll remember, "She was always making jokes, was flippant, obnoxious, loud." I have to be constantly prepared. If you're black, there's no one on your side fighting for you, sticking up for you.

In many minority cultures, the family is traditionally a tighter, more supportive unit than in the majority culture. The African American, Asian American, or Latino medical student often has a viable safety net and cheering squad:

> My grandparents on my Mom's side were my role models. They were farmworkers in Chile and had very strong values. My grandfather never completed third grade and my grandmother never completed fourth grade, yet they both could read and write. They didn't see themselves as handicapped by their lack of education. They viewed formal education as one avenue and learning through life as another avenue. My grandmother was excellent at math—she could do computations in her head—and knows history like anyone I've ever met. It was good to feel loved and cared for by other people who were just like me.

Pyskoty, Richman, and Flaherty assessed black, white, and Hispanic medical students according to psychosocial assets and mental health status, first on entering medical school and then a year later. Entering minority students were found to have these advantages: greater social supports, higher self-esteem, lower anxiety, and more internal locus of control. After one year, however, they showed higher anxiety than whites and increased external locus of control. Students in both minority groups showed increased distress and decreased feelings of self-efficacy. Minority students often feel competing demands between their kinship and friendship ties and work needs. Majority students are generally socialized to focus more on their own needs and inner resources and to look to others for support less often.[40]

One reason to facilitate minority medical education is to provide medical services for medically underserved communities. A Chicano student recalled, "Minority admissions interviewers will ask right off, 'After you finish medical school do you plan to practice in your community?' " He reported, "I'm most definitely going back—that is the main reason I am here. Our services are desperately needed in our own communities where the white doctor won't go."

Many minority students share this goal. They see wrongs to be righted—members of their community may not be receiving the same quality of care as patients from the majority culture. A third-year student recounts:

> Black patients are very vulnerable. They often don't have any insurance and they're at the mercy of these [medical] residents. During the Los Angeles riots, I cared for two patients with very different needs. One African American patient had a very painful sickle cell crisis. The other, a well-developed, well-nourished white man was in no pain but may have had a myocardial infarction. The team discharged the African American patient early and without adequate pain management because they thought he might sell it out on the streets. If it had been my decision, I would have let the other guy go. I think black people need more representation. This is where I want to work, with people who have no insurance, those I can fight for.

According to a spokesman from the National Medical Association, an organization of black MDs, black physicians are at a distinct advantage not only in relating to but also in interpreting a black person's complaints because of shared life experiences. "There is a significant impact in having similar experience [if quality care is a consideration]."[41]

An African American doctor agrees:

Being a black woman is the most positive aspect that I can bring to this institution for patient care. The empathy and compassion and understanding I have for them is a big part of my job. When I interview patients and prepare them for surgery, it is 100% easier for me than my white or black male colleagues. I'm able to extract information from them that they wouldn't tell anyone else.

Interviews with 18 Latina physicians committed to work within their culture show a similar attitude. One explained:

I have been through it myself. As I grew up, I received services at county facilities. This gave me an insider's view of patients that others don't have and I'm more sensitive to their needs. Rather than saying to a patient, "Get on this diet" without considering how much it will cost them, I can counsel them more sensitively about how to change their dietary habits and eat foods that more likely fit their customs.

The ability to translate helps the young physician feel important. "I've become a hot commodity," one noted:

I have a marketable language that puts me in demand. In my residency training, most of the attendings didn't speak Spanish, and they looked to me for information and help. Eight out of 10 times a diagnosis is based on obtaining a complete history. Understanding ethnic and cultural backgrounds of the minority patients has served me well.

On the flip side, the bilingual physician can feel exploited: "It becomes a burden when you're walking down the hall and someone grabs you to explain something to a patient you don't know anything about. They don't realize that it takes a lot out of my day."

A Latina physician viewed her minority status as a source of compassion and tolerance. "I think being a Latina has allowed me to see things from different points of view. I can identify very well not only with my Latin patients, but with others as well. Whether they're low-income whites, blacks, or Latinas, I have a view into their worlds." Another Latina reported that her background gave her perspective: "It's given me a sense of appreciation for what I have. Sometimes my classmates feel that their life will be destroyed if they don't get the grades they want, but I realize that such little things aren't important when compared to the bigger things in life."

Students With Physical Disabilities

It is estimated that more than 1,000 physicians in training have physical or learning impairments. Such students point out that they don't want pity, just the same opportunity as others. They don't want others to say, "Oh, here's this disabled student. Let's treat him with special care."[42]

Medical students are not immune to health problems. Terry Loder, a recent graduate of the University of Utah School of Medicine, had her matriculation delayed by two years due to a brain tumor. "I hadn't shown any symptoms until I had a grand mal seizure at a concert," she said. After surgery and chemotherapy she returned to school only to experience more seizures and a second tumor. Now she will use what she learned from the experience in her neurology career. "Being here and being healthy is probably the greatest gift I could have and the rest is just icing on the cake," she said at graduation.[43]

Like all aspiring physicians, the physically disabled face the challenge of admission to medical school. A medical student in a wheelchair tells about an application interview:

> Because I considered ———— to be a progressive school that strives for diversity, I was shocked by my experience there. The interviewer didn't ask about my academic achievements, interests, or future plans. Instead, he was concerned about my health insurance and the financial ramifications for my family. He even asked if my parents liquidated their assets to pay my medical bills. I had heard that some schools conduct stress interviews so I played it cool and answered the questions without expressing my anger or disgust. The interviewer had the audacity and ignorance to ask me specifically, "Medical education is very expensive and a lot of work. Will you be alive in four years to benefit from your education?" I restrained my initial response to verbally put him in his place, and responded, "Yes, my prognosis is excellent." He then asked if I would be willing to obtain a letter from my doctor stating my prognosis for the admissions committee. I was so stunned I didn't know what to say.

This student was accepted at another school. Three years later, reviewing his academic file for his residency application, he found letters from his personal physician to the assistant deans updating them on his medical condition—an appalling, perhaps illegal, but certainly blatant disregard of personal, confidential material.

Dr. Thomas Strax, a physician with cerebral palsy, is medical director of the John F. Kennedy Health Center in Edison, New Jersey. He stresses "that no otherwise qualified applicant should be denied admission based on physical and psychological characteristics."[44] AMSA established a task force in 1994 to improve conditions for disabled students. Headed by a hearing-impaired student and another with cerebral palsy, the task force planned to provide a forum and basic support for medical students with disabilities. It also hoped to educate medical students and personnel in this area. As Strax points out,

> Most people think suffering a disability is isolated, but guess what? At some point in their lives, 50% of everyone—you've got a 50-50 chance—will have a chronic disability that will handicap them or prevent them from getting into places they want to be and doing things they want to do. And you won't be prevented because of your disability, but because of how others perceive you. We all need to be activists for better access—and I don't mean just ramps.[45]

A Latina medical student was hearing impaired for years, relying on a hearing aid and lip reading. In her senior year of college, her hearing failed altogether.

> I thought it was my hearing aid, my battery. No! It was me! I had progressive sensorineural hearing loss. I really wanted to graduate, and I thought medical school was history, I'll admit. I trained to read lips better. I learned sign language. I went back to class and they gave me oral interpreters and note takers.

In addition to managing her studies in a whole new way, she had to deal with her feelings about her deafness.

> I knew I could stay there and feel sorry for myself or go forward and see what happened, and I went on and things went very well. I was graduating! So since I was doing well, I decided to take the MCAT, then I applied to medical school and got accepted. But even now I am still making adjustments to being deaf, really accepting that I'm deaf.

Most of the medical school faculty were facilitating. "Professors have come up to me personally to ask me to let them know if they can help me in any way." One professor opposed her, however:

> One teacher was very tough. She asked the interpreters who they were and what they were there for. She was very strict with me. One time, during an exam, we had to identify something on a slide. She would tell the other students to find another slide or a better spot, but she ignored me and just walked off. When I went to talk to her, she looked at the interpreter and asked, "What did she say?" I spoke up, "I can talk for myself, I will repeat it if you need me to." Finally, I talked to the dean. After that, she saw I was doing well and became more friendly.

A young woman orthopedic surgeon, crippled from childhood because of polio, commented that the most difficult part of her training was not the physical demands or the pain in her joints. Rather, it was, "the emotional drain of having to prove myself over and over again."[46]

You may even be challenged by other physicians who have disabilities, as this student was:

> A family friend who practices cardiology told me that he didn't think I could be a physician if I didn't wear a prosthetic leg, not because of aesthetics but because he didn't believe I could move fast enough. He was paralyzed by polio and requires the use of Canadian crutches to ambulate. I am much more agile and quicker on my crutches than this man is on his own. His preconceived notions of wearing a prothesis is an example of biases which exist in the medical profession even among disabled physicians.

Ways of coping with a disability are as varied as the students themselves. The first two years of medical school went well for this physician, but when she began her clinical rotations, her body lagged:

> I faced an on-call night. I began to realize that I had organized my life in such a way that I was nearly always able to get the eight to nine hours of sleep that I desperately needed to refuel my energy and relax my aching muscles. Three days after my on-call day-night-day, I was still feeling physically incapacitated, unable to concentrate very well . . . and beginning to feel hopeless and depressed. I asked the Assistant Dean of

Students for a modification of my call schedule. He asked me if perhaps I wanted to consider withdrawing from medical training—a shocking question to which I responded with a resounding "No." Although his retort was, "I was hoping you would say that," he also suggested that I strongly consider a medical subspecialty that would be less taxing.

In a less physically rigorous residency, psychiatry, her health returned. Looking back, she admits she isn't sure she would do it all again. And yet, she knows her struggles have made her a better psychiatrist. "I know what it means to suffer, to experience that internal heart-rending anguish, the conflicts over one's inner drives and external reality."

A pregnant anesthesiology resident trained in an earlier day said her attending

> was adamant that anesthesia could only be given standing; it was like painting, he said. Sitting wasn't allowed. This became a problem for me with long cases, due to my polio weakness. When I became pregnant, the situation became acute. I had to sit and didn't see why you couldn't. I began sitting for most of the anesthetic, much to everyone's horror. No one had dared to this before. I proved you could, and have spent many years sitting throughout cases, including intubation. This was the first step towards my now permanent philosophy, "Work smarter, not harder."[47]

Now, most anesthesiologists routinely sit.

Some physicians find their disabilities are assets. One paralyzed doctor said he "learned from his own experience what patients really need from doctors." He speaks openly with his patients about his paralysis and finds it makes them more at ease with their own medical problems.[48]

A family practitioner who was born profoundly deaf teaches and does research at a university. His impairment—he doesn't consider it a disability—made him work harder, he says. "It's made me more tolerant, more perserverant."[49] Dr. Spencer Lewis, who formed a national organization for handicapped physicians (the term at that time), summed it up this way:

> Just because one has a handicap, one doesn't automatically become mentally deficient. So much goes into what I call the complete physician; a certain amount of education, compassion, experience, good sense. Some people have particularly sharp or well-honed senses. You've run into the

person who can hear the murmur that nobody else can hear! Just losing one or two faculties does not mean that the whole person is worthless. I want people to be more sensitive and aware of people with handicaps—and of the knowledge that they too can be good physicians.[50]

Gay and Lesbian Students

Although homosexuality is more widely acknowledged and accepted than in the days when the *Diagnostic and Statistical Manual* of the American Psychiatric Association (APA) listed it as an aberration, gay and lesbian students still meet with discrimination in most segments of society. Medical school, with its notorious "good old boys, boot camp mentality," is no exception. One student recalled applying for a psychiatric residency and receiving an unexpected rejection letter. "I later found out from others on the committee that I had been selected, but the committee chairman had rejected me because he wasn't comfortable having a gay resident."[51] One gay student recounts two incidents with intolerant fellow students:

> A Muslim student with whom I considered myself on very friendly terms told me that he felt homosexuality was incompatible with civilized society and I should change. He went into this whole history about how the gay community was irresponsible and hedonistic. This same student was dating a girl who converted to Islam, and she started wearing the hood. Our class has a little newsletter, and someone had made a quip in the paper about how this individual had gone into hiding under the hood. The Muslim student was very offended by that comment and went up in front of the classroom to accuse the person who wrote that of being prejudiced. He accused the class of being intolerant to Muslim students and said that they were going to be forming a Muslim support group. And that we have to be more accepting of other people.

Another student was overtly hostile.

> When a classmate of mine asked me if I was gay, I told him, "Yes," I was, and I hoped he didn't have a problem with that. Although he said he didn't have a problem with it, he started making comments to some of the other students behind my back. Then, one day at the cafeteria, I was sitting with friends and this same guy disagreed with something I said. After

my friends left, he called over two students I didn't know and in the middle of the cafeteria he announced to them, "Did you know that this guy here is gay?" He said it very loudly, with his finger pointing down at me. I was very insulted, very angry.

Then, the next day in class, they were announcing class officers for different groups on campus and they asked if there were any representatives of MEDGLO [the gay and lesbian medical student group]. I was sitting halfway across the room—and he leans out of his chair and yells to me, "Hey, do we have any MEDGLO representatives in our class." He was essentially trying to degrade me as an individual. He was also making sexual comments to the women in our class. So I went to the dean of the school and told him this individual was acting very inappropriately. I said, "This is simply intolerable. I don't care what his feelings are, but while we're here at school, while we're colleagues, he needs to learn what is appropriate to say." And the dean totally agreed and called him in. But of course, this guy told all his friends that I had done this horrendous deed, and I felt repercussions for what I had done.

House staff and attendings sometimes make critical comments about homosexuals, unaware that they are talking with one. "I hate f———," a surgeon said to a third-year lesbian student on his way to evaluate a man with perirectal abscess. "I really hate f———, that's why I could never do colon rectal surgery. I would have to deal with these people all the time." Keeping silent during this incident, the lesbian student later commented, "I don't think that 'straight' people understand what it means to have to hide or be silenced. . . . All lesbians and gay men have to do it at one point or another and hate themselves for it."[52]

"It's a disadvantage to be different and to feel different," said a second-year medical student:

The medical world is small; it's like a club and people talk about each other. If you're different in any way you experience negative exposure. Medical student classes, a weird group of overachieving, anal people who are under a lot of stress and time pressure, can be very supportive or very judgmental. There's a lot of hazing that goes on, some of it very subtle. So you always feel you are being subjected to some kind of nasty prejudice and you wrestle with whether you want to be out or not out, quiet or stand up for what you believe in—whether it's anybody's business or not. It's a disadvantage to be different in any way.

Gay and lesbian students are often unwilling to reveal their sexual orientation because of possible social stigmatization and discrimination.[53] They long for social support, friendship, and social opportunities. "It has always amazed me that people could hate me so intensely for loving a woman who loves me back," said a medical school graduate."[54]

Those who hate are not even involved. For decades society has tried to cut a deal with gay people. "Stay closeted, don't make us look at you and acknowledge who you are, and we will leave you alone." This is not the case, and in fact, we are not left alone. Anti-gay laws and enforcers enter our homes and places of congregation and arrest, harass and even kill us for nothing more than loving each other. It's not fair or American or moral.

What do gay people want? I cannot speak for all of us, but I can speak for me. I want not special, but equal rights, meaning the right to be protected under the law as other minorities are, not persecuted by the majority because I am different.[55]

Two issues are of particular relevance to gay and lesbian medical students: whether or not to be open about their sexuality and the impact of AIDS on the homosexual community. Now the two are related: "Whether to be open is a very personal decision. With AIDS a lot of people are going to be looking at gay physicians with suspicion—will I be getting AIDS from my physician? The general community assumes that a lot of the gay community is HIV positive."

Many gay physicians keep their identities hidden because of this concern. "There are a lot of gay physicians, but most of them keep it quiet. People don't know." Those who choose to be open must be prepared to deal with the consequences. "If you do decide to be open, you have to be strong enough to carry through with it, not to be intimidated or ashamed," one said.

The homosexual students sometimes find themselves in a position to educate their classmates. "I've had other students come up to me very curious," a gay student explains:

Several have asked me, "What does this mean?" They've never interacted with openly gay or lesbian people. They ask questions like "Haven't you ever been interested in women?" "What is it you want out of life?" "What does your future look like to you?" I don't have a problem with that.

Students who interact with an openly gay or lesbian person generally find that homosexuals are "no different than anyone else. Knowing openly gay people at medical school 'takes the mystery out of it,'" said one observer. "I will definitely feel more comfortable with my gay patients as a result . . . and I have learned that I can't assume anything about my patient's sexuality."[56] "Prejudice and hatred are harder to perpetrate when the victim is someone we know or love," notes Lydia Vaias.[57]

Like members of other minority subcultures, the homosexual student may plan to treat medical problems specific to that community—in this case the prevalent AIDS crisis:

> I envision myself treating predominantly AIDS-related conditions. And it's going to require a strong physician, because all or most of your patients are going to die. The patient is also going to be very dependent on the physician, not only to be very up-to-date with medical treatments that are changing constantly, but also to be emotionally supportive, both on a personal level and with significant others that may be involved. In addition, the physician has a responsibility to educate the community. AIDS touches the gay physician on a very personal level as well as on an academic level.

A family practitioner notes that the referral service of the Gay and Lesbian Physicians of Chicago (which lists 75 doctors) receives 50 to 100 calls monthly from gays and lesbians looking for "doctors who are affirming of their lifestyle." "It's not that the patients bear a prejudice towards heterosexual doctors," he says. "It's their fear of how doctors respond to them, because most gays and lesbians have experienced bias in some form, subtle or overt." Gays and lesbians constantly face physicians who don't understand their health needs. Because discussion about sexual behavior is so limited in medical school and many doctors have never had a human sexuality course, many physicians are unfamiliar with sexual diseases and don't ask about personal habits. Patients aren't comfortable with physicians whom they need to educate initially or doctors who are uncomfortable dealing with gays and lesbians.[58] A third-year woman student reports,

> Some residents are surprised at the questions I've asked gay men about their sexual activities. I explain to them that as their medical provider, I have to know their risk factors. For example, contracting HIV differs

when one receives or gives anal sex. The residents just ignore such topics and never ask. But it is an educational opportunity for both me and the patient.

Like other minority students, the gay or lesbian medical student may find strength in being different. "You bring a different perspective," a lesbian observed:

> You are more able to understand people who are different, and most people who are sick are different from young white males in their 20s who are robust, healthy, and intelligent. A lot of patients are indigent, miserable, poor, and lots of other horrible things. I think it makes you a little bit more understanding of where they're coming from.

One student remarks, "It's not all bad to be different when you go to medical school. And it's important to trust some people who are straight, because you're going to be working with them." Another student advises,

> Remember that there's more to life than one's identity as a member of the gay community. Don't be totally absorbed in your sexual orientation. There's a thousand and one other issues which you'll be dealing with as a physician. Your sexual orientation is probably just a small part of a bigger picture.

Older Students

At one time, very few people over the age of 30 went to college, let alone medical school. In fact, medical school applicants past their 20s were actively discouraged. When she picked up the forms to apply for medical school in 1980, an older woman who is now a physician was told, "We don't take anyone over 28." She commented: "In that day, young was better, white was better, male was better, science major was better. But over the years, we've learned that these superficial things don't make a doctor. To be a good doctor, you must be a good human being, a person who has good character."

Affirmative action has made age an unacceptable admission criterion, and the number of older students in the country's medical schools is slowly increasing—from 5% in 1975 to 12% in 1994. Some schools, such as Michigan State University College of Human Medicine (which recently admitted a 59-year-old), prefer older students. "We really like older applicants," says the director of admissions. "The older students bring realism and a tremendous experiential base. They've already gone through the hard knocks that it takes to become a professional, and they are realists about their medical degree."[59]

A woman who graduated from medical school in her 50s describes her decision to attend medical school:

As a child, I wanted to be a doctor. But I married young and had children. Our son was in medical school, partly because of my interest in the field. I called him and asked him to see if there was an age limit. He said, "A few years back there was a woman who was 50 when she graduated." I said, "Okay, I can do that."

Another physician was a teenage mother and a high school dropout. Widowed at age 19, she worked for 12 years for an ambulance service before she began college. Then, supportive people, noting her obvious talent, encouraged her to enter medical school. "Sometimes it doesn't seem like it's really true," she said at graduation. "I think that if I can get through medical school, then people can do just about anything."[60]

Unfortunately, some older students encounter discrimination and report discouraging remarks at their medical school interviews:

The interviewer said that he would give me the highest rating he could and although I would be great for the school, he knew I wouldn't get in. I asked him why and he said, "Because you are so much older and have that much less time to actually function as a doctor."

Rejection can be devastating, as one applicant relates. "I have a Coast Guard license; I fly aircraft; I started a company—and all of a sudden I can't make the grade here." He felt like a failure for the first time in his life. Like this individual, second-career students pursuing medicine have often been successful in previous careers. "It's not that they have failed and then decided to pursue medicine," Owen Peterson, the assistant director at Harvard, says. "They just found that their work was not fulfilling."[61]

A judge retired from law at age 54 and traded his gavel for a stethoscope.[62] "The law treated me well, but I wanted to be a doctor ever since I graduated from college," he explained. "But I had no premed training and nobody to counsel or encourage me to go into medicine so I went to law school instead."

This 31-year-old woman student explained the advantages of her age and experience:

> I saved enough money to go to medical school without getting into massive debt and working exposed me to a lot of different people. I've had more chance to experience life and have some fun. I've worked in the hospital and know how it works and how to get along with the people who work there. Although I feel a little isolated from my younger classmates, I still go to their parties and have lots of friends who are only 21 or 22. I feel that my classmates accept me and I can act as silly as they can. Still, there is no one there my age that I could ever possibly date. But I don't have time to date in medical school anyway.

For the most part, older students encountered very little discrimination, but exceptions occur, as this student recalls: "[One] doctor took an instant dislike to me simply because of my age. On my evaluation he wrote, 'This is a mature woman who is slow.' I am *not* slow!" She complained, "I'm glad he put the word 'mature' because it shows where he's coming from. The other team gave me honors." A resident on her first rotation was openly hostile:

> He told other people that he didn't think it was fair that I was there, that I was taking up space that a younger person could have used who could have practiced longer. I tried not to let it affect me. Then, on the last day, I went up to discuss a patient with him. And I had learned how to present a patient. He was sitting there looking very casual, and he said, "Okay, just give me the bottom line." I thought that meant, "Let's not have a whole formal presentation; just tell me what is wrong." I told him what I thought was wrong, and he jumped up—he was about 30, six foot five inches tall, real skinny—and he started yelling at me. "What's wrong with you?! Don't you know how to do a correct presentation?!" He didn't give me a chance to answer and backed me up through the clinic in front of the nurses, shouting at the top of his lungs, "You have a test tomorrow! How are you going to pass it?! You don't even know how to write a prescription!" (The very first day I hadn't known how to write a prescription and had asked one of the other residents how to do it.) He was screaming

at me and all I could think was, "I know they're not going to put that on the test."

Fortunately, she added, sometimes her age earned her added respect. "Most of the people I dealt with were younger than my own children. They treated me with more respect than they would other students." A younger student remarked, "Older students are definitely good role models. They just seem more 'put together' than I am."

Older students sometimes feel that they need more time to study. "I have to take more time to study at my age than I used to 30 years ago. I think I have fewer neurons than I used to. They say you lose 10,000 a day. It takes me longer, but once I learn it, I learn it well." Stamina may be a problem. Another student acknowledged, "I know that I don't stay up and study as late as many other students—I don't do all-nighters. I usually do get 7 hours sleep at night. I get enough done so that performance-wise, I've always been in a comfortable position in exams."[63]

The physical rigors of medical school weren't a problem for this older student:

Staying up all night was hard at first. But you get used to it. What you're doing is extremely interesting and busy. The hard part is getting through the next morning. But you can't go home to sleep, you have to go home and study. When my feet would hurt, or my back would get tired, I would never say anything, but generally one of the other students would say, "Oh, my back is killing me." I would think, "Oh, this is normal. I can live with it." . . . The whole four years of school, I averaged about five hours sleep a night when I was not on call. Maybe older people don't need as much sleep.

She compared notes with another older student: "I talked to an intern in her 40s. She said it's not the physical hardships that bother her so much as not seeing her family."

Family is clearly impacted when an older woman goes back to medical school. One student commented that her husband would "get very upset and touchy because things weren't being done for him anymore; rather I expected things to be done for me. It was a real role reversal." Other ties may also be weakened. "Friends would call and want to chat, and I'd have to say, 'Sorry, I really need to get studying.' So they stopped calling."

Insights: Staying Centered
Bernard Virshup, MD

I like to give the Jungian Types test to my first-year medical students. It makes them more aware of the diversity of the human experience. There is an infinite variation in the way each individual person can respond. No one ever is "typical." We each have a style that is uniquely us. Each person can say to the world, "Yes, this is the way I am. I like being this way."

This test gives students an opportunity to look at the variety of people around them, without idealizing anyone (since each has weaknesses) and without deprecating anyone (since each has strengths). More important, it allows them to accept their own strengths and weaknesses, without self-aggrandizement or self-deprecation. It allows all students to feel realistically good about themselves.

You will be surrounded by students and teachers who think their way is the right way to be and to do things. Students have favorite living styles and study habits; teachers imply they know what you must do to be successful. Each believes his or her way would be best for you. What can you do with all these opinions? Can you take what fits, perhaps experiment a little, and finally fashion a style that is unique to you? Probably the single greatest challenge you will face in medical school is remaining inner directed, staying in charge of yourself, deciding for yourself what and how much you should study, how much time you will give to medicine, how much time to take for yourself and others.

What can you do before going to medical school to prepare to handle other people's possible negative opinions of you? Here are some things you can do to practice:

- Pick out an article of clothing that reflects your mood and wear it without considering how it looks, whether it is in style, or what people will say.

- Drive on a freeway at five miles below the speed limit (not in the fast lane, please). Can you set your own speed and keep to it? Or do you have to keep up with the traffic?

- When you pass a beggar on the street, look at him or her, make eye contact, smile, and don't give any money. Do you feel like a terrible person? Can you be manipulated by needy, helpless people? Are you forced to be "good" by your own internalized need for approval? Or are you a good person because you choose to be?

- Take half an hour every day to do something for yourself that you will continue throughout medical school, something that will be non-negotiable and will take precedence over anything else that is demanded of you.

Notes

1. AMSA Advertisement. 1986, July-August. *The New Physician,* p. 44.

2. Calmes, Selma Harrison. Forthcoming. "From the Far Side: Women in Anesthesiology 1966-1996." In B. Ray Fink, ed. *Careers.*

3. Walsh, M. R. 1977. *Doctors Wanted: No Women Need Apply: Sexual Barriers in the Medical Profession, 1835-1975.* New Haven, CT: Yale University Press.

4. Buck, Genevive 1994, June 12. "Mirror images. More Patients Looking For Doctors Who Reflect Their Concerns." *Chicago Tribune,* Section 5, p. 4.

5. Associated Press. 1995, May 31. "Medical Schools Note a Gender Shift in First-Year Classes." *Chicago Tribune,* Section 1, p. 3.

6. Nelson, Harry. 1992, May 20. "Will Female MDs Bring Women's Touch to Healing? (growing numbers of women physicians mean change)." *Los Angeles Times,* p. A5.

7. Paxman, Sue. 1994. "Adding Another Floor." *Exponent II,* 18(4):2.

8. *Ibid.*

9. Clark, Elizabeth M. 1994, April. "Women in the Health Care System. Part 2: As Physicians." *Journal of the Medical Association of Georgia,* 83:195-198.

10. *Ibid.*

11. Burke, Edmund C. 1992, September. "Women in Medicine: A Promising Future, Despite Challenging Past." *Minnesota Medicine,* 75:5.

12. Asta, L. M. 1995, March. "Halting Harassment." *The New Physician,* pp. 31-38, p. 31.

13. Fugh-Berman, Adrianne. 1992, January 20. "Tales out of Medical School (women medical students, sexism at Georgetown University Medical School)." *Nation,* 254(2):37-41.

14. Coombs, Robert H., and Hori Hovanessian. 1988, January-February. "Stress in the Role Constellation of Female Resident Physicians." *Journal of the American Medical Women's Association,* 43:21-27, p. 22.

15. Rush, Shelby. 1992, October. "Everyone Is Suspect." Letters in *The New Physician,* p. 3.

16. Rush, Shelby. 1992, September. "Usual Suspects." *The New Physician,* pp. 15-16, p. 15.

17. Gross, Edith B. 1992. "Gender Differences in Physician Stress." *Journal of the American Medical Women's Association,* 47(4):107-111.

18. *Ibid.,* p. 110.

19. Klass, Perri. 1996. "The Feminization of Medicine." In Delese Wear, ed. *Women in Medical Education: An Anthology of Experience* (pp. 81-94). Albany: State University of New York Press, p. 91.

20. Asta, *op. cit.*, p. 33.

21. Clark, *op. cit.*, p. 196.

22. Clark, *op. cit.*

23. Milani, Laura. 1995, March. "Going the Distance." *The New Physician,* pp. 47-52, p. 49.

24. Clark, *op. cit.*, p. 197.

25. Milani, *op. cit.*, p. 48.

26. Baker, Lawrence. 1996, April 11. "Differences in Earnings Between Male and Female Physicians." *New England Journal of Medicine,* 334(15):960-964.

27. Tesch, Bonnie J., Helen M. Wood, Amy L. Helwig, and Ann Butler Nattinger. 1995. "Promotion of Women Physicians in Academic Medicine. Glass Ceiling or Sticky Floor?" *Journal of the American Medical Association,* 273:1022-1025.

28. Buck, *op. cit.*

29. Milani, Laura. 1995, March. "Women's 'Ways' of Doctoring." *The New Physician,* pp. 20-21, p. 20.

30. "COGME Report Calls for Better Training Opportunities for Women." *Public Health Reports.* 1991, January-February, 111:3-4.

31. *Ibid.*

32. Crandall, S. J, R. J. Volk, and V. Loemker. 1993, May 19. "Medical Students' Attitudes Toward Providing Care for the Underserved: Are We Training Socially Responsible Physicians?" *Journal of the American Medical Association,* 269(19):2519-2523.

33. Heins, M., J. Hendricks, L. Martindale, S. Smock, M. Stein, and J. Jacobs. 1979, November. "Attitudes of Women and Men Physicians." *American Journal of Public Health,* 69(11):1132-1139.

34. "Fewer Minorities Apply to UC Medical Schools." 1997, June 16. *Los Angeles Times,* p. A16.

35. Tschida, Molly. 1996, May-June. "The New Physician's 17th Annual Minority Admissions Score Card." *The New Physician,* pp. 24-25, p. 25.

36. Wallace, Amy. 1995, November 19. "Figuring Out Who to Let In." *Los Angeles Times,* pp. A1, A30; p. A30.

37. "Minority Admissions Scoreboard." 1993, March. *The New Physician,* p. 14.

38. Campos-Outcalt, Doug, Paul J. Rutala, Donald Witzke, and John Fulginiti. 1994. "Performances of Underrepresented Minority Students at the University of Arizona College of Medicine 1987-1991." *Academic Medicine,* 69:577-582.

39. Fadem, Barbara, Mark Schuchman, and Steven S. Simring. 1995. "The Relationship Between Parental Income and Academic Performance of Medical Students." *Academic Medicine,* 70:1142-1144.

40. Pyskoty Charlene E., Judith A. Richman, and Joseph A. Flaherty. 1990. "Psychosocial Assets and Mental Health of Minority Medical Students." *Academic Medicine,* 65:581-585.

41. Buck, *op. cit.*

42. George, Steven C. 1995, January-February. "Ready and Able." *The New Physician,* pp. 13-18.

43. Gehrke, Robert C. 1996, May 19. "'Real Life' Produces Great New Doctors." *Salt Lake City Deseret News,* Section A, p. 20.

44. George, *op. cit.,* p. 16.

45. George, *op. cit.,* p. 18.

46. Beyette, Beverly. 1989, May 28. "A Surgeon—Against All Odds." *Los Angeles Times,* pp. 9-11, p. 10.

47. Calmes, *op. cit.*

48. Mack, Ruth A. 1990, March. "A Dream Disabled?" *The New Physician,* p. 6.

49. Anstette, Patricia. 1994, June 13. "Deaf Doctor." *Chicago Tribune,* Section 5, p. 4.

50. Holmes, Michelle D. 1983. "The Life and Legacy of Spencer B. Lewis." *Harvard Medical Alumni Bulletin,* pp. 52-55, p. 55.

51. Roan Shari. 1994, July 5. "Growth—and Growing Pains—for Association of Gay Doctors." *Los Angeles Times,* pp. E1, E5; p. E5.

52. Tinmouth, Jill, and Gerald Hamwi. 1994, March. "The Experience of Gay and Lesbian Students in Medical School." *Journal of the American Medical Association,* 271(9):714-715.

53. Townsend, Mark H., Mollie M. Wallick, and Karl M. Cambre. 1991, June. "Support Services for Homosexual Students at U.S. Medical Schools." *Academic Medicine,* 66(6):361-363.

54. Vaias, Lydia. 1995, November. "Setting the Record Straight (President's Column)." *The New Physician,* p. 32.

55. Townsend, Wallick, and Cambre, *op. cit.,* p. 32.

56. McGrory B. J., D. M. McDowell, and P. R. Muskin. 1990. "Medical Students' Attitudes Toward AIDS, Homosexual and Intravenous Drug-Abusing Patients: A Re-Evaluation in New York City." *Psychosomatics,* 31:426.

57. Vaias, *op. cit.*

58. Buck, *op. cit.*

59. Yoo, Teresa. 1995, September. "Dreams Deferred." *The New Physician,* pp. 23-27, p. 24.

60. Gehrke, *op. cit.*

61. Yoo, *op. cit.,* pp. 24-25.

62. Moss, Brenda. 1995, November. "Courting Medicine." *The New Physician,* p. 43.

63. Yoo, *op. cit.,* p. 25.

Second Year

Do I Really Want to Do This?

When my Mom calls and asks about the weather I tell her, "I don't know; I don't go outside."

—Second-year medical student

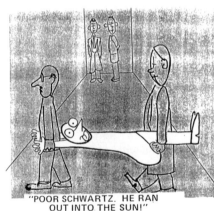

"POOR SCHWARTZ. HE RAN OUT INTO THE SUN!"

After a year of pressure and emotional turmoil, you may question your career decision to become a doctor. Many second-year students seriously consider dropping out. "Rampant depression struck our class—more so than the first year—because we could see what we were up against." Second-year courses seem even more difficult than those in the first year, and you must study to pass Part I of the medical boards at the end of your sophomore year. Add to this the accumulated affects of a devitalized social life and it is not surprising you may feel emotionally exhausted. Still, there is a sense of achievement and progress, for you have survived what many regard as a highly challenging ordeal.

Transformation

During the second year, the most stressful academically, you will begin to perceive yourself differently. Your confidence will increase and you will start

---

The cartoon above is used with permission from Charles F. Johnson, MD.

to take a more active role in directing your own medical education. You will be more vocal in objecting to what you perceive as unfair or unnecessary and more assertive with faculty members to get the information and assistance you need. Best of all, you will develop a clearer sense of what is important to learn instead of just what is necessary to pass exams. "The first year, you're more oriented toward passing and getting the material down. The second year you're more oriented toward what you're going to have to know for the patient's sake," said a sophomore medical student.

Although second-year tests may occur less often, they are just as threatening. But if you are like most students, you will take satisfaction in the realization that you are more skillful at knowing what it takes to pass, more critical in your judgments, and more selective in your responses to demands on your time.

As you proceed through your second year, you may notice changes in yourself. Changes will almost certainly occur, products of your growing maturity, of the confidence you gain as you "learn the ropes" about the medical center, and of the realization that clinical responsibility comes next. Toward the end of this year, you will have increased exposure to patients, mostly in the role of observer. You will be encouraged to ask questions and form opinions, and you'll see actual clinical situations. Course emphases will change, focusing more on diseases and abnormal states than on the pure science of the first year.

Gradually, you will begin to assume—or you will be offered—the role of a neophyte member of the medical profession. You may be enthusiastic at finally getting down to the business of medicine or alarmed at being expected to act on so little knowledge and experience. Intellectually, your reaction will most likely be to concentrate your efforts on "learning things that will help you to help other people." If you are like most students, you will find your second year a sobering experience.

As a second-year student, you will still confront an overwhelming amount of material to learn in a short time. Yet, you will probably have more confidence in yourself, if for no other reason than that you've "made it this far." "Now that I've got a year behind me, I know I can do it if I just apply myself." "By now, you figure, 'I passed last year and I can pass this year.' That fear is out of the way." "I, personally, and the whole class seem less uptight."

Class Work

As a second-year student, you will spend less time deploring the lack of clinical relevance in materials presented and correspondingly more time anticipating your next year of full-time clinical service. The first year's academic agonies come into perspective. "We had the background the first year; in the second year we begin to apply it at *least* a little bit." The change in attitude toward your course work will reflect not only curriculum differences in the second year but also alterations in your own perceptions. "The worst class this year is better than the best class last year." "This year's been more in the nature of what I'd like to study—more functionally relevant material. Most everything we have seems to be worth learning." "The courses themselves are more stimulating." "Pathology is the nitty-gritty, the stuff we really have to know." "All the stuff we learned in freshman anatomy comes together second year in physiology." Even pharmacology, a course more oriented to basic science and usually taught by PhDs, may seem exciting. "Here's a disease, and here are the symptoms, and you put together the knowledge with the problems. You may not come up with a solution, but you come up with a guideline or direction. It isn't all seemingly irrelevant, intellectual abstractions."

It is to be hoped that the fact that not everything can be learned and retained will be less threatening to you the second year than the first. As one student put it, "Students habituate to the futility of hoping to understand everything." And optimism gradually replaces stoicism. "Nobody expects you to learn it all. It's mainly a foundation you're building." "You become more adept at handling the vastness of the material and picking out some points." "You learn about a particular configuration and say, 'Gee, that was important to understand,' and you know the reason because someone may be coming into your office in a while with that particular problem." "Instead of school, grades, and homework, medicine becomes a way of life." "Academically, I've become more selective. I study what I think is important and I do more outside reading on my own than I ever did before. Medical journals are becoming more and more interesting and understandable."

Complaining about the faculty, curriculum, and classmates may help you relieve pent-up pressures and maintain emotional equilibrium. You'll notice an increased feeling of achievement and progress and a desire to make the most of every opportunity. "We have only four years here and there's only so much we can learn in this amount of time. I want to make sure I'm doing as much as I can in the time I have." "Last year, I had to adjust to the fact that I was covering about as much in a day as I'd covered in a week in college. This year, I had to readjust to covering as much in one day as I did in two days last year."

Chances are that you will see yourself as more serious as you get closer to the reality of becoming a doctor. You will then "begin to feel the position you are going to assume in society." "You feel a lot of responsibility, and that has a sobering effect." For some, this weighty responsibility seems to be coming on too soon. "You feel like you're supposed to be equipped to make medical decisions after your sophomore year. But right now you know a little about a lot; you have a smidgen of many things but don't feel really confident in bringing it all together." For others, the real clinical experience can't come soon enough. "The academically oriented ones are fearful and the clinically oriented ones are ready to shout with joy!"

Faculty

By the second year, you will probably feel that the faculty's attitude toward your class has improved considerably. You will be more receptive, owing to your greater grasp of fundamentals. As for the faculty, "They're more comfortable with second-year students. They can discuss things they're more interested in." You will sense that faculty members feel they can afford to give more of themselves because you've begun to prove your mettle. "They have a lot invested in you by the time you've got a year behind you, and they'll think twice if your performance is bad—they'll ask why." "Almost everyone feels that anybody who gets this far should get through."

Another important difference in your mutual regard is that more instruction is now offered by physicians. "The teachers this year have more clinical experience; they're exposed every day to what's important to a clinician." "The MDs realize, 'These are our fledglings,' but the PhDs regard their lectures as their duty to us." "The clinical faculty tends to regard us as members of the club; PhDs teach us only because it's their job."

Although you may have felt as a first-year student that the faculty had little desire to do anything but subjugate or embarrass you, in the second year you are more apt to sense benevolence and to react accordingly. "This year the general atmosphere is, 'Well, you're going to be a doctor soon and we're here to help you.' That's my own feeling. If I'm going to be a doctor, I'd better buckle down and learn." "The teaching staff seems to respect us now. They lecture to us as though we are really going to become physicians. I really appreciate that. They tend to give us little pearls of wisdom and insight into what we'll encounter in practice."

The psychological distance from the faculty lessens, and your sense of participation increases. Greater emphasis is placed on what you observe, and you are encouraged to ask questions and draw conclusions. "I don't think we have any professors this year who haven't cracked jokes. It may seem like a small thing, but it's really relaxed the class. We feel that we can approach most of the professors; we don't fear them as we did last year." "They bend over backward to get their points across. After all, to keep medical knowledge going they've got to teach what they know to somebody else."

If you are a woman or from a minority culture, you may yearn for mentors of your own gender or background. It is difficult to feel part of the "club," to possess a sense of identity or belonging, when the "medical fraternity" consists primarily of Caucasian men. "I have been frustrated in my search for an adequate role model, a professor who is a female physician." "As a female student, I've had few contacts with women MDs. It would help my adjustment if I could relate to women faculty members or even speak to women who have passed through this stage and returned to the outside world."

Fortunately, things are changing. More junior faculty members are women, although department chairs and the upper bastion remains overwhelmingly white and male. In addition, most of the younger faculty are accustomed to women as colleagues, which diffuses tension between genders. Male physicians married to female physicians tend to be very sympathetic to women's issues as well.

Hospital Hierarchy

As a second-year student, you will feel a greater sense of identity with the medical center. "The freshmen are the babes—the ones you wean. We are walking." Although you may not have a sense of belonging on the hospital floor, you at least can see where you will fit in. Sometime during the second year, you will observe and interview patients, although you will actually have little clinical responsibility regarding the day-to-day realities of hospital life. As one student explained, "A sophomore is a potential that hasn't yet caused an accident."

During this transitional period, you will begin building relationships with hospital personnel. "On the totem pole of the teaching hospital, the sophomore medical student is second from the bottom—only freshmen are lower." According to another student, this assessment may be overly optimistic: "In my experience, third-year students are on the bottom of the totem pole. First- and second-year students have not yet earned a place on it."

Many students at this level readily acknowledge the greater practical competence of nurses and paramedics and realize they have much to learn from them. "I don't mind being lower than the paramedical people. I've got to learn from somebody." "In a lot of respects, most of the paramedical staff are more competent in clinical work than we are. All we know is from books right now." "Nurses are often wary of medical students until they feel comfortable that a particular student knows enough not to harm their patients." "You can't tell nurses anything about hematomas or injections—they know it all. You can't tell chemical technicians about blood chemistry because they know more than you ever will." "Most of us are totally ignorant about how the hospital really works."

Despite the disparity in practical knowledge and skills, some of your second-year classmates may assume a superior role, relying on their educational background and future physician role to afford them status. "In private, each person figures he's pretty low in the pecking order because he doesn't know anything practical. But when we all get together, the attitude is, 'Boy, when we get up on the floors, we're going to be fairly high up relative to the paramedical staff.'" "We get our status from the doctors and the faculty. They show us what our worth will be by taking the time to teach us." "The more you know, the higher the ranking you get."

For those students who assume superiority, the subservient role they must continue to play rankles. "Most frustrating to students are the medical techs who teach us in the spring. Some of them put on a pretty superior attitude." "This is their big moment of glory, and they can't help having a holier-than-thou attitude. It's like they're saying, 'You dummy, can't you even stick a needle in a vein?' Those less caught up in the status game, however, find the relationship less hostile: "I've encountered a cooperative spirit among paramedical staff and the medical students."

Student Togetherness

As you advance through school, you may sense a new relationship with classmates and other members of the medical community—a feeling of kinship, of being in it together with a shared purpose, direction, and motivation. You will alter your perceptions of your classmates and of the nature of your own interdependency. "We understand each other better now." "Everybody knows where everybody else stands, so there's more rapport than last year." "You're out to do the best you can, not to prove yourself better than others." "We seem to respect each other's differences, and in that sense there is more unity." "We have arguments, but we're much more of a class now." "We're united in one respect; we have a common goal."

Although you will probably continue to rely heavily on your classmates—"Another medical student is really the only one who understands"—

you will begin to feel more independent, more in control. You will still view grades with apprehension but feel less competition with classmates. "We are pretty loyal to each other. If one of us finds out something that will help the rest of the class, we go around sharing it. People are not as apt to keep things secret for their own advantage." Competition, when it does occur, takes on a friendlier tone. "There are just a few people who are so bright they leave the rest of us behind. The remainder of us are kind of along in the middle."

When a classmate is in trouble, you may perceive a collective threat. For instance, a female student questioned a male professor's gynecological procedure and he responded defensively, "Well, look, Blondie." At that point, "the entire class came to my defense, arguing with him and pointing out that he had no right to talk to a professional person like that."

Perceived differences between classmates tend to blur. Increasingly, as you move through school, you will only dimly recognize the individual differences that once seemed so important. "I don't see groups as I did last year." "There's none of this hot factionalism like there was last year." "The big North-South division has kind of gone, and there are few, if any, militants." "I don't think there are cliques like last year; it seems more like one big group doing the same thing at different times." Preconceived images give way to a common status: physician-to-be. "Well, I just see them in the same boat that I'm in. All of us are striving for a specific goal—to become an MD."

In spite of distinctions that never disappear (e.g., the ultracompetitive types who simply gear up to battle for residency slots), most of the stereotypes, divisions, and labeling fade. "Everyone seems more alike now than in the past. I used to classify them as playboy type versus studious type. Now, I think everyone is becoming more of a professional type—the type you would think of as a doctor."

As you move from the classrooms, labs, libraries, and study halls into the world of hospital wards, you will begin to see yourself as part of a larger system, in which you and your peers have more in common with one another and with the faculty than you do with others outside the realm of medicine. And sometimes this will even include your family.

Hurdles

In spite of this heightened perspective, some second-year students wonder if they made a mistake in choosing a medical career. The price—chronic fatigue and anxiety—may seem too high.

The Boards

Passing Part I of the national boards looms over the second year. Success can open the doors for the immediate future, such as getting into a competitive residency. Most medical schools end classes several weeks before the boards to give you time to review the material from your first two years. For some, the boards provide an opportunity to showcase all their hard work; for others, they constitute the greatest career hurdle to date. Some wonder if high scores are more indicative of a good science student than a good future physician.

The board exam places enormous stress on you because failure to pass after three attempts shuts the door *forever* on practicing medicine in the United States. Most medical schools will not allow you to continue clerkships or go on to the third year until you have passed Part I of the boards; some students are "yanked from the hospital floors" as soon as grades are received. The sudden disappearance of a few colleagues from your summer clerkship can sober you—it could have been you. But almost all those who fail seem to have had difficulties throughout the first two years' classes. Some students use this exam as their watershed experience, allowing themselves to finally succumb to the "weeding out" process. Part II of the boards is taken at the school's discretion any time after the second year. Part III comes after graduation when the trainee is enrolled in an internship program. Parts II and III are more clinically oriented than Part I and passing rates are much higher. "It is said," a third-year student remarked, "you study two months for Part I, two days for Part II, and bring a pencil to Part III."

Financial Strain

Financial concerns and problems affect academic performance, social life, and self-esteem. "One of the big things for me is that I'm 24 years old and still not financially independent. I'm still relying on my parents." Fadem, Schuchman, and Simring found that parental income correlates with student scores on the Medical College Admission Test (MCAT) and U.S. Medical Licensing Examination (USMLE) Step I, particularly for minority women.[1] They postulate that those with parental resources can more easily deal with unexpected expenses and buy supplemental goods and services.

Students from economically disadvantaged families, particularly women, may be employed outside of school or may use some of their school financial aid to assist their families. Finances may be their biggest stressors in medical school. "I'm financing my education on faith and a shoestring. My reserves are completely exhausted this year, and I'm in debt. I'm very uneasy about it because all these debts have to be paid back, and I'm just getting deeper in." "I'm getting pretty old. I hope I don't resort to picking an easy specialty just so I can get out quickly to earn a living." From a second-year single mother, "Even at this point, I don't know if I will be able to complete medical school because of financial hardships. It's a month-by-month sort of thing. I'm never quite sure how I'm going to make it."

Social Life

Financial concerns can also hamper social life. "I hate asking my dates to pick me up or to come over here to watch TV. I feel cheap—but then again I feel really bad when I think about how much money I'd go through in a year on dating." And there are other impediments. Even those actively opposed to the "all work and no play" maxim find medical school a *major* disruption in pleasurable outside pursuits:

> While I was studying for the boards, I was in the library full-time; I went when the doors opened and left when they closed. I met some Russian physicians there who were also studying for the boards and we became friendly. How sad it is to have to meet people like this!

Married and single, students feel they are "getting stale" or "becoming warped." "Medicine is 99% of your life. You're not able to keep up with the outside world." "I see myself in a rut walking from home to school and back home again." "Studying all the time can make you feel so alone." "I fear that I'm becoming more boring by the day." "Being cut off from everyone else makes for bad doctors, I think." "I did manage three dates during the second semester, but the rest of the time I ate, slept, and studied. It tends to make me wonder why I am continuing in medical school."

When they do take time away from studies, students tend to feel worried and guilty. "You feel really bad when you talk to somebody who has been gunning it all week for a test and you played golf or went out on a date. You *are* here to learn, and maybe you ought to be in the library instead of running around." "There are only a few times during the year you can call your own, just to relax with a clear conscience." "You tend to forget all other people when you are under pressure. You think you are more important than they are and then you feel guilty for allowing yourself to lose perspective and be overcome by the system." "I get awfully depressed and sometimes don't feel like talking. I'm getting more pessimistic, less talkative, less willing to express my opinion." "I have less patience with my wife—don't try to understand her problems."

Students, especially those who have been active in athletics, complain, "You're always sitting. Nine months out of the year I'm in school and miss the recreation and exercise I need. At the end of the evening, I drag myself home all pooped out. I get physically run down." "I'm concerned about it from a health standpoint." "This attitude of 'total consumption' by school is unhealthy and needs to be dealt with from the start of school." "I still don't understand why studying health requires sacrificing one's own." "How can you create health care providers in an unhealthy atmosphere? It's like training nuns in a brothel."

Psychic Stress and Coping

The stresses of medical school accumulate. In a study of medical student stress, the psychologist Thomas Wolf concludes, "It appears as though graduating medical students are worse off psychosocially than when they entered as freshmen."[2] An earlier study found anxiety among first- and second-year medical students higher than that of psychiatric patients.[3]

The American Medical Student Association Foundation sponsored a national conference titled Medical Training: A Matter of Survival? The keynote speaker, DeWitt C. Baldwin, Jr., scholar in residence at the AMA, reported on a survey of 580 medical students: 87% had been publicly humiliated, 81% had been verbally assaulted, 55% had been sexually harassed, 37% had been assigned tasks for punishment, 27% said someone took credit for their work, 19% had been racially harassed, and 18% had been hit or pushed. In addition, Baldwin reported that 70% of the residents in his study noted impairment in their colleagues, including alcohol and drug abuse, sleep impairment, and emotional problems.[4]

Typically, women are more at risk than men because they are caught between traditional and contemporary gender expectations and, as a rule, receive less social support. Women are more apt to define themselves in terms of interpersonal relationships, to feel responsible for relationship maintenance, and to be susceptible to others' demands.[5]

Informal support groups buffer against stress. You may, for example, confront the conspiracy of silence by acting as mentors to first-year students:

Everyone displays such bravado that it's rare for anyone to admit to feeling overwhelmed or depressed—feelings that everyone has. When I talk to younger classes, I really try to dig down and reveal my own struggles, because I think everyone needs to know that even the students who appear most competent go through times of doubt and sadness, loneliness and fear.

"Sometimes the people who are most relaxed in class are 'secret gunners' at home. Don't be fooled; it's hard for *everyone.*"

Organize your schedule to accommodate health-enhancing activities. One student limited her study schedule with a stopwatch. She resigned herself to whatever grades she received and spent "guilt-free time" with her husband or on other activities after filling her quota of study hours. "I'm sure if I had bumped it up to seven hours per day on the weekends my grades would have been better, but my sanity would have suffered. Those hours were all I was willing to give, and a 3.5 GPA was fine with me."

Some students successfully lobby the faculty and administration for well-being committees to sponsor health-enhancing activities. When AMSA distributed a well-being survey to its 140 chapters, 40% responded with only half (50%) reporting that their schools provided well-being programs.[6] In a similar survey of medical schools in the United States and Canada, Thomas Wolf and Philip Scurria found a lower number—just over 30% of schools provided health promotion and wellness programs.[7]

Some schools offer support services such as individual counselors or small discussion groups. "Freshman year we had a group that met once a month at a professor's home for dinner and a discussion. It was a great sharing experience!" "There are social support groups and various counselors to help with stress now."

Wolf's research showed that medical students' emotional and physical health tended to suffer from the stresses of medical training, so he and his colleagues organized a well-being program at Louisiana State University Medical Center in New Orleans.[8] A well-being handbook given to the incoming first-year class presents general principles of well-being and describes program components. The handbook lists aerobics classes, small discussion groups led by third- or fourth-year student advisers, progressive relaxation techniques, meditation, self-hypnosis training, visualization, time management techniques, and nutrition.

The UCLA Student Well-Being Committee sponsors a variety of sub-committees directed by third- and fourth-year student volunteers. At first-year orientation, students receive materials describing wellness enhancing opportunities; in small group meetings led by second- and fourth-year students, they are encouraged to enroll and volunteer for leadership positions to plan specific activities. One of the most popular is a series of dinner seminars held in faculty homes. Other seminars and discussion groups focus on substance abuse awareness, coping skills, and cultural diversity. Some program activities include Practice at Improving Relationships for couples (PAIR); a parents group; City Explorers (tours of the area for out-of-town students); Over-26ers for older students; ethnic groups for Chicano, black, and Asian American students; and an organization for gay and lesbian medical students.[9]

This committee also sponsors service opportunities. These include the Flying Samaritans, who periodically help staff clinics in rural Mexico, and Big Sibs (second-year students who volunteer as informal counselors for incoming first-year students). The committee also publishes a student newsletter, called "911"—a survival guide based on the wisdom of second-year students.[10]

Medical training is admittedly a stressful experience, but medical students, faculty, and administrators can make well-being a priority at their school. Hall and Miller state, "There are considerable data that physicians are at greater risk for psychiatric illness, substance abuse, and suicide than the general population."[11] Make a point to maintain your own physical and emotional health.

Insights: Relaxation
Bernard Virshup, MD

You may sometimes become distraught to the point where you will find it difficult to concentrate and may even feel helpless and hopeless. Many have found it useful to take time out; and meditation is one way of doing this. Meditation, a time-honored way of inducing an altered state of consciousness, creates calmness and serenity.

Herbert Benson, a researcher at Harvard Medical School, recognized this calming effect as the opposite of the fight-or-flight response, the body's natural reaction to stress.[12] He dubbed this state "the relaxation response." People who regularly elicit the relaxation response become resistant to the effects of the stress hormone, noradrenaline. It takes greater amounts of the hormone to produce the increased heart rate, blood pressure, and other changes that characterize the stress response. When Benson studied meditators in his laboratory at Harvard, he found that as the volunteers shifted from simply sitting quietly to meditating, their breathing and heart rate slowed, metabolism slowed, oxygen consumption dropped, and brain waves took on patterns associated with rest and relaxation. Blood levels of lactate—a chemical associated with anxiety—dropped precipitously. Benson believes that meditation consists of two elements: the silent repetition of a sound, or mantra, to minimize distracting thoughts; and passive disregard of intruding thoughts, followed by a return to the repetition. The same elements are present in religious and cultural practices the world over. In a series of studies, he showed that the repetition of a single, neutral word, such as "peace," could produce these physiological changes and overall sense of well-being.

Many people evoke the relaxation response best if they focus on a word or phrase that has a special meaning—perhaps something from their religious tradition—rather than a neutral word. Anyone who is interested in trying the relaxation response can begin to practice it easily. You need to find 15 to 20 minutes in your daily schedule, such as before breakfast, when your time may be free of all distractions. Practice every day until you see if it's helpful to you. (Practicing twice a day can be even more effective.) You may begin to feel calmer after just a few sessions.

Here is the set of instructions used at the Harvard University Mind/Body Medical Institute:

- Pick a word or short phrase to focus on, perhaps one that's rooted in your personal belief system. If you're not religious, you might choose a neutral word or phase like "one" or "love." If you're religious, consider a phrase from your tradition.

- Sit quietly in a comfortable position, close your eyes, and relax your muscles.

- Breathe slowly, in a comfortable rhythm, repeating your focus word or phrase silently as you exhale. As you do this, don't worry about how well you're doing. When other thoughts come to mind, simply say to yourself, "Oh, well," and return to the mental repetition.

- Continue for 10 to 20 minutes (pick a length of time beforehand and stick to it). You may open your eyes occasionally to check the time but don't use an alarm; it's too jarring.

• When you finish, sit quietly for a minute or two, first with eyes closed, then with eyes open, to smooth the transition to ordinary life.

Many thoughts may come into your mind as you are meditating. You may think, for example, "This isn't working." O.K., that's just a thought; note it and return to your mantra. The key is not to try to meditate but to just allow the process. It will happen by itself; you can't make it happen. Just keep returning to your mantra. If you become aware that your limbs are heavy and your thinking slowed down, you may think, "Oh, I'm meditating! "O.K., that's just a thought, too; note it and return to your mantra.

The following meditation exercise may help you center yourself when you have been knocked off center. You can record it and then listen to yourself as you play it back.

A Centering Exercise

There are two different ways of seeing the world. One way is to identify and name. For example, take a moment to look around the room and notice what you see. Sometimes, after we have been in a place for a while, we tend to stop being aware of things. See how many objects in this room you can name. Now, shift to another way of seeing the world. Look at it as an artist or photographer might—not as a set of objects but as shapes, light and dark, patterns—how would it look as a piece of art through a viewfinder?

Now, close your eyes, and do the same thing with your ears. Listen for sounds you can identify. What do you hear? Voices, air conditioner, doors closing? Now, shift to another way of hearing. Listen to these sounds as if you were a composer, and you are going to include these sounds in your new, modern symphony.

Keep your eyes closed, and pay attention to what your hands are touching. Identify what they are touching. How do you know that? What is the sensation in your skin that lets you know what your hands are touching? How does the touch get translated to a signal your brain can identify? What is that sensation?

Do the same with your body posture. You know what your body posture is. But how do you know it? What is the sensation in your body that lets you know where it is?

Now, do the same with your arms and legs. Of course, you know where your arms and legs are. How do you know it? What is that sensation?

You know you are breathing. Of course, you are. But how do you know it? What are the sensations that let you know you are breathing?

Besides breathing, your heart is beating. Can you be aware of that too?

Quite a lot is going on in your belly. Can you feel your bowel rumbling?

Somewhere in their body, most people have a place they consider more them than anywhere else; a kind of center. Some people feel it in their head, or chest, or abdomen. Where do you feel this center?

Your center is a place you can feel safe, relaxed, secure; a place you can enjoy; where you can feel good about yourself, where you know you are O.K. Stay there for a little while. It's a good feeling. It is a place you can always go, any time you wish.

Now, slowly, come out to the real world. Look around. Experience other people. Enjoy the world. But know that any time you wish, you can return to your center and feel safe and refreshed.

Notes

1. Fadem, Barbara, Mark Schuchman, and Steven S. Simring. 1995. "The Relationship Between Parental Income and Academic Performance of Medical Students." *Academic Medicine,* 70:1142-1144.

2. Wolf, Thomas M. 1994, January 28. "Stress, Coping and Health: Enhancing Well-Being During Medical School." *Medical Education,* pp. 8-17.

3. Vitaliano, P. P., J. Russo, J. E. Carr, and J. H. Heerwagen. 1984. "Medical School Pressures and Their Relationship to Anxiety." *Journal of Nervous and Mental Disease,* 172:730-736.

4. Baldwin, DeWitt C., Jr. 1992, March. "Dignity and Respect: Essential Conditions for Student Well-Being." Keynote presentation at the American Medical Student Association Foundation National Conference *Medical Training: A Matter of Survival?*

5. Dickstein, Leah J., Judith J. Stephenson, and Lisa D. Hinz. 1990. "Psychiatric Impairment in Medical Students." *Academic Medicine,* 65:588-593.

6. Baldwin, *op. cit.*

7. Wolf, Thomas M., and Philip L. Scurria. 1995. "A Survey of Health Promotion Programs in U.S. and Canadian Medical Schools." *American Journal of Health Promotion,* 10(2):89-91.

8. Wolf, Thomas M., Howard M. Randall, and John M. Faucett. 1990. "A Health Promotion Program for Medical Students: Louisiana State University Medical Center." *American Journal of Health Promotion,* 4(3):193-202.

9. Coombs, Robert H., and Bernard Virshup. 1994, January 28. "Enhancing the Psychological Health of Medical Students: The Student Well-Being Committee." *Medical Education,* pp. 47-54.

    10. *Ibid.*
    11. Hall, F. R., and M. J. Miller. 1994, January 28. "Health Policies and Proce-
dures for Medical Students at U.S. Medical Schools: A Progress Report." *Medical Education,* pp. 26-32.
    12. Benson, Herbert. 1975. *The Relaxation Response.* New York: Avon.

CHAPTER 5

Relationships

Am I Married to Medicine?

My wife complains that I don't treat her as well as I do my patients: "You're friendlier to your patients than you are to me." But when I get home, I'm so tired and irritable I don't even want to talk to her at the dinner table.

—Senior medical student

The "Outside World"

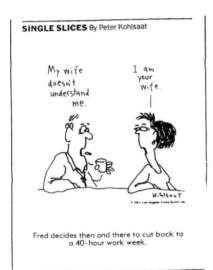

SINGLE SLICES By Peter Kohlsaat

Fred decides then and there to cut back to a 40-hour work week.

However time consuming medical school may be, there is, of course, a world going on outside. If you're like most students, you will identify with the profession when you interact with "outsiders"—those relatively uninformed about your day-to-day life in medical school—and they'll view you with pre-existing attitudes about "doctors." This can afford a strong element of ego gratification, especially in contrast to the ego battering that goes on in school. "There's no way a human being can enjoy being told he's stupid, no way he can enjoy doing scut work, being the lowest man on the totem pole." Out of school, a medical student has an opportunity to be somebody unique. Many students bask in the glory of "doctor-to-be." "It's nice to have people look up to you and say, 'She's going to be a doctor!'" "When you go home, you're the only medical student in the crowd, and people really respect you. You feel you have to play the role of physician."

Some students feel their own accomplishments have already set them above other people. "I see myself on a higher level than graduate students because medical school is so much harder." "PhDs use the title 'Doctor,' but when people call someone 'Doctor,' they usually mean 'Doctor of Medicine.' I don't think most PhDs would correct that impression."

This role playing can have a down side. "I never thought it would get to the point where somebody would be visiting and my mother would try to get some medical advice out of me, but it did!" "My parents look up to me and ask a lot of questions I don't like answering. I want to tell them to go to consult with a doctor." "It's frustrating because after the first day of medical school everyone assumes you know everything about diseases. When I tell them that I won't study that for a couple years, they look at me like, 'Well, what kind of doctor are you going to be anyway?'"

In recent years, many students have become sensitized to the changing public image of doctors and their "divine right" to enjoy high esteem in the community. "I think the doctor is falling off the old pedestal and being trampled underfoot." "The public is just hostile enough to take the doctor to court when there's the least little question." "They're beginning to know more and question their doctor."

However you view yourself or are viewed by others, in terms of your status as a prospective MD, you'll find that you are different and set apart from others. You will often be lonely. "I've gotten the idea that a medical student is not like anyone else." Few will fully understand the pressures you experience, share your changing perspectives on humanity, or be able to empathize with your problems. You will be cut off from many of the routine pleasures that you enjoyed as an undergraduate and that your nonmedical friends engage in.

Dating will pose special problems. If you are married, you may encounter unique adjustment problems. Financial dependency and debt will probably be a fact of your life long after most men and women your age are paying their own way and enjoying financial security. Depending on your own personality and adaptability, these problems can assume overwhelming importance or can be dealt with on a philosophical level. "There's the course, there's the obstacle. Now, we've got to get around it."

Loneliness

Although as a medical student you are more likely to be independent, you will probably be afflicted by a sense of unwanted isolation at some times in your training. Most students do feel lonely, even during the clinical years. "I feel very isolated, socially and culturally." "Even when you work in a hospital with hundreds of people, loneliness is a factor." "I feel like I'm at the other end of the world from everybody." Clinical rotations in a variety of hospital settings break up close friendships made in the first two years. "Since medical students and residents all work on rotations, you are with the same people for a month at the most. You work night and day with them, get very close, and then rarely if ever see each other again." "My intern told me he likes having med students around because it gives him company. He too feels alone most of the day."

Living arrangements often perpetuate this physical separation. Particularly in off-campus medical centers, many single students live in virtual isolation. "Loneliness is one of the big things now that I live by myself, and it can be real drastic." Some seek familylike arrangements to relieve the pressure of being alone. "I room with another student, and we live with a couple who are real nice to us, they sort of mother us. If you were by yourself, with nobody to talk to, you'd go out of your mind." Others prefer greater privacy but confess to missing companionship. "My landlady goes to bed at 8:30 every night, and I can't watch TV, can't do this and that. In that little room with me, myself, and I, we don't get along so good all the time!" "I live by myself. I'd like someone medical to live next to me, just so I could discuss this stuff with them." "It gets me down every once in a while, just to walk into that apartment with nobody there."

Alienation

Going home for a vacation affords students, especially single ones, relief from the isolation of medical school. "I'm very close to my family and a very select group of friends at home, and it's hard for other people to fill in." Sometimes, parents and friends can provide much-needed enthusiastic reinforcement. "My folks are gung ho all the way. I can do no wrong in medical school." A few students, especially those whose parents are in medicine, even find a new basis for mutual appreciation. "My father's a doctor, and I talk to him more now. Since he's experienced it, he's sympathetic, and I can identify with him a little more." "I go home on Sunday and go on rounds with my father. I'm finally able to talk with him."

But for others, going home simply increases their sense of remoteness:

I went home one weekend on a Friday afternoon after a frustrating physiology exam. The next day my mother told me she couldn't even talk to me that night; I had been impossible. I'd never before come in contact with anybody outside medical school during exam time. It felt kind of funny.

"When you're studying 24 hours a day for finals you can't even make normal sentences."

When you go home and speak to someone not in medical school, they expect you to say it's fine, you really like it and are enjoying it immensely. But occasionally, somebody perceptive wants a true answer so you tell them it's lousy, that you don't like it a bit. It really puzzles them, because it's something you've wanted to get into since high school.

"When it's all added up, I feel that I don't fit in the medical environment and no longer fit comfortably outside of it either."

It's possible that you'll find your parents' perceptions of your new status—or even your own status perceptions—set you further apart from them. "My father was on cloud nine when I got accepted and he's a tad surprised when somebody asks me a question that I can answer. To him, a doctor is a distant person who knows an awful lot, and he gets surprised—'Hey, my son is really doing this.'" "My parents now have a doctor, not a son." "I'll be the first doctor in our family—they put it on a much higher pedestal than I do." "My Mom always says, 'My daughter the doctor.' One day, I'm gonna say, 'What about your daughter the teacher and your son the businessman?'"

If you depend on your parents for financial assistance, this may be an additional source of strain between you. "I've always been very close to my father—a little less so as I've become older. I think I resent more and more that he's my bread. He finances my tuition, car, and other personal expenses. He and my wife also split the groceries, rent, phone, and electric bills."

If you are already uncomfortable with your dependency on parents, a comparison with friends and acquaintances who are pursuing a more "normal" life course can be unsettling. "All my friends are in Manhattan, living in their apartments and running around. I picture what they're doing compared to what I'm doing and it makes me feel a little jealous." "My friends who are not in medical school are financially independent, but they are still incredibly supportive of me—they know I cannot afford much and always insist on paying when we go out." "Even at the end of medical school, your income is meager, and if you go on to specialize, here you are at 35 years of age before you can go out and make any kind of living." "After eight years of higher education you are only worth a little over minimum wage as an intern. Entering-level food service workers make a dollar less an hour than medical interns."

Students' personal struggles are often exacerbated because they are kept under wraps, due in part to the medical school stigma against expressing one's emotions:

I had six deaths in my family, plus my parents divorced during my first two years of medical school. I felt like I was going crazy. My parents were calling me daily to complain about each other. Then, with everyone dying, I had the cadaver experience and I needed to sort through my feelings about death. I felt there were no other students I could talk to—they all seemed to come from perfect, stable homes, with both parents MDs, no money troubles, etc. I later learned that the reason it seemed that way was because everyone was keeping their mouths shut and dealing with their personal problems either like me or in psychotherapy.

Although most students experience alienation, loneliness, and other personal struggles, faculty and advisers typically ignore these personal aspects of being a student. Just as the impact of abrupt status change and adaptation to stress are left to the individual student to work out, so is the adjustment to alienation from family, friends, and the outside world.

This apparent institutional indifference to the emotional side of medical students may be perceived as another of the deliberate, if unacknowledged, processes of socializing doctors. Because they are cut off from other people, medical students are forced to become increasingly self-reliant and to gain personal fulfillment solely from their medical experiences. Willingness to accept loneliness and alienation and to persevere become additional criteria for the physician-in-training. Some students argue that these lonely challenges help them become "better and stronger" people. Development of cynicism and detachment may be the price many pay to become a physician, however.

Students have become increasingly more vocal about the need for outside involvements and show less willingness than their predecessors to settle for the "introverted medical student" role. They form activist organizations, voluntarily participate in community health programs and summer health projects, and pressure medical school administrations to become more involved in community outreach programs. "It's important that you have something going on on the outside so that you don't get completely lost in just books and the loneliness." Moreover, as one student pointed out, "Social activism is not just therapy for lonely people; our society really needs it!"

Forming Couples

Predictably, the loneliness, alienation, and frustration of young adults in medical school are often compounded by romance relationships—or the absence of them. Depending on you and the location of your medical school, you may expect some disruption in your normal dating pattern.

Dating

First the good news. Some single students, especially men, find that medical student status enhances their desirability as dates, and some even claim they date more in medical school than they ever have before. "Some wear their white coats and name tags everywhere." "The way society looks at doctors—and here I am going to be one—helps with the dating situation." "The guys in our class are sought out. The girls from the sororities come right across and camp in our library to meet them and say, 'Well, here we are.' And that's valid because the guys don't have time to go looking." "Some men even organize supper clubs to further enhance meeting women." "I hop, skip, and jump all over the cafeteria and make passes at every female I see. It's not hard to get one to go out and raise some hell." "I look at it like this. I've gotten this far. I'm going to be a doctor. I've always put off social interactions for school. Now, it's time to pick up the slack in that area."

Now the bad. Some women are reluctant to date medical students. "It's hard to ask a girl just to come over and be there. Medical students have the reputation of wanting company only for sex." Managing sexual urges can be a problem. "Most medical students, when they get out on a date, move pretty fast. They want to make up for it all in one night." "When you *do* get a Saturday night off, that's the time for wild partying and getting as much in as you can. This is the time to skip the preliminaries and get down to action." Shortage of leisure time, unpredictable schedules, physical exhaustion, and general tension all contribute to a common plight summed up in the term "deferred sexuality."

Single students differ in their personal standards of what is an appropriate outlet for sexual drives. For those who choose not to abstain until marriage, the aforementioned problems are compounded by the absence of a readily available partner. "A lot of unmarried students practice abstinence because there's just no time." "You can't devote all the time and effort to taking a date out, getting to know her, for just that one instant. Therefore, I think a lot of single students lean toward masturbation." Then, there's the situational approach: "It makes a difference how close to exams you are and how sexually inhibited you are at the time."

Students of both sexes may feel too pressured by their course work to even want to date or don't enjoy it when they do go out. "Dating isn't as much fun as it used to be." "A woman who decides on a medical career should know that her dating won't be too keen for 8—or maybe 20—years." And still others complain that their dating life suffers from a lack of a "suitable" partner. "It's awkward to tell a guy you're a med student—'Oh no, she's smart!'" "One problem is a lack of females of the college type." The problem is tougher for women students, even on a college campus. "You can't walk around the hospital wearing a sign: 'Looking for a date.'" "The guys in our class are *much* more socially immature than a comparable group of men in the general population, and the undergraduates are too young and just aren't interesting."

Many students are reluctant to date someone within their class, although reasons vary. "Nursing and paramedical students solve a basic ego need that my classmates can't solve for me. It's nothing new when I tell another med student what I've done all day. They've done it, too." Female students report, "The guys in our class just don't pay any attention to us nor consider us as a possible social group for any kind of interaction." "I think it's because you're stuck looking at that person for the next four years if it doesn't work out. The class gossips a lot, 'Oh, what happened there?' If it doesn't work out and you don't remain friends when it's over, then you've got a lot of tension."

And there are also reservations expressed about dating others within the medical center. For male students, nursing students, nurses, and auxiliary staff represent the most readily available source for dates, but many resist, alleging that nursing students are "too young," nurses "too old and bitchy," and all others "not intellectually stimulating." Perhaps more to the point, *all* of them are reminders of the hospital environment. "The nursing students are cute as they can be, but there's a generation gap there." "I don't want to come across a girl I'm dating in the course of the day, have to eat with her in the cafeteria, and walk with her down the hall." "When I'm off, I like to be off. I don't want to talk about medicine."

Choices at the hospital are slimmer for female students and the problems considerably different:

We aren't treated completely as the young medical *male* student—everybody sort of looks at us and says, "All right, this is a woman, and we're going to test her to see if she operates well." You can't be hustling or flirting at *all*. A couple of us have dated doctors in the hospital, but you really have to make a definite effort to maintain a very professional attitude.

"If you're not flirting and trying to interact, then they're turned off. You're not going to be asked out by someone who thinks you act cold."

. Female medical students also have an image problem. "The guys think we're strange. Plus, as a group, we're pretty hard nosed." Men who have traditional views expect to be the primary breadwinners, with their wives in supportive roles. They are usually not comfortable with assertive women and may be intimated by women who make more money than they do. Women who study medicine are usually much more assertive than their female counterparts. This may make it more difficult for a female medical student to meet men and maintain a long-term committed relationship. "If you are a guy with a beeper on your belt, you'll have a flood of women around you immediately when you go into a bar. But if you're a woman with a beeper, the guys will be suspicious, 'Why do you have a beeper? Are you a drug dealer or something?'"

Some students choose informal cohabitation, which offers many of the emotional and physical comforts of marriage without the risks and obligations of a permanent commitment. One student put it bluntly: "I'm having a girl move into my apartment for the last three months I'm here, sort of a live-in buddy and date. She looks on it more or less as a trial marriage, but I look on it as a way to prevent loneliness, to have somebody here."

Mate Selection

In their mid to late 20s, with a lifetime of school behind them, many single students want more than casual relationships. And most aren't looking merely for compatible partners who can accept or enhance the medical school experience but for the "ideal doctor's mate," someone who will complement their medical career. As one student expressed it, "Nobody wants to work just for himself. You wonder if you'll ever find the right person to marry." Others admit a craving for companionship, stability, financial and emotional support, and (among male students at least) a desire to be relieved of household chores. "I'm not eager to get married, but I see so many people obviously happy, and sometimes I feel a little lonely." "It'd be nice just to have someone there when you get home," said a woman student. "It's horrible to say, but my friend and I always joke about how nice it would be just to have a body to hold." "It would help to have somebody who could fix a meal and iron a shirt and clean up after you," a male classmate remarked. And when you're married, "You don't have to take a date out for a show or dinner. You can stay home and watch TV."

Some female students regard their male classmates as basically insecure in their sexual identity and perceive their marital choices as influenced by this insecurity. One woman explained, "The male medical brain maintains a dichotomous view of women: Wives are to be loved but not taken seriously as creative people, intelligent wage earners; female colleagues are respected but not lovable—not taken seriously as females—just 'one of the boys.'" "I don't want to be married to an MD," another woman commented. "When would we see each other?"

Some men support this point of view. "I'd like to marry someone who thinks along my ideas, who is intelligent, and who has enough sense to let me play the masculine role, even though she may be smarter than I am in half the things." "I want to marry someone who isn't extremely domineering; I want to be the domineering one in the household." Other men emphatically do *not* fit the sexist mold. "The woman I date is a sophomore medical student, and we've talked about marriage. I'll be away for a year in internship and she can't come with me. I don't expect her to quit her job and follow me—I'd be disappointed if she did." And some students' logic transcends mere sexism: "I hope to marry a girl who's rich!"

Students who arrive at medical school engaged or with an "understanding" may encounter new strains on their relationships. If the partner is close at hand, the medical student may find that time restrictions, focus on studies, and other school-induced tensions frustrate both of them. "Medical school has had a bad effect. During my senior year in college, we were together every day." Conversely, the partner may be far away with relative freedom to enjoy life. "I have a girlfriend who goes to school pretty far from here, and she does a lot of running around. I want her to, because she's kind of young, but I feel myself relying on her a lot more as my decisions here get tougher."

On the other hand, "There have been many successful relationships and marriages born in medical school, so if you want to date, there are plenty of opportunities." One student tells about his wedding to a classmate:

We had our pathology final on a Friday and the next day we got married. We were up at the alter, lighting the candles and standing together listening to the organ play and she is asking me how I did on the pathology final—you can see it on the video camera! It looks like we are whispering sweet nothings, but we are talking about the pathology exam. We hadn't seen each other—not until at the alter.

Marriage

For many students, marriage provides financial security they couldn't otherwise attain. "Most of us who are married live off our spouses' salaries and get tuition from another source. Those who are unmarried have to obtain living money as well as tuition money." "Before I was married, I was dependent on my parents and I didn't like that. *Now,* I'm dependent on my wife." "My training is paid for with loans and my husband's salary. I'd like to be able to pay him back some day." "If I hadn't gotten married, it would have been a huge burden on my parents."

But financial strains are still present, and both spouses are aware of the sacrifices involved. "My wife and I were eating at the hospital for two or three months because it was cheaper than eating at home." "We haven't done a lot of socializing this year for two reasons. One is time, and two is we've been a little short on funds."

Emotional Support

The value of a supportive spouse cannot be overemphasized. "It really helps to have a supportive and understanding partner who can put up with the unpredictable schedule, fatigue, and crankiness that I go through." "With the pressures you're under, having a wife is just tremendous." "We're both students and we understand each other very well when we are tired. I was worried about our marriage after hearing all the statistics on poor physician relationships, but we have had no problems. We owe our successes to having one another for support." "My husband has always been very supportive. He likes the fact that I have strong career interests and I'm pursuing something that I feel is important."

A longitudinal study of male medical students I conducted with Fawzy Fawzy showed that compared to their unmarried counterparts, married students are generally more relaxed, better motivated, and less likely to be depressed and anxious.[1] I also found that when single students marry during school they cope more successfully than they did while single. Married students can go home to supportive companionship and a healthy outlet for their sexual urges and feel that *who* they are matters as much as *what* they do.

Female medical students and physicians typically receive less support and face greater demands at home than men. "Women take care of more things than men do," one woman observed. "The two guys I work with have wives who do everything around the house for them. One guy has never done laundry in his entire life! His wife does everything—pays the bills, schedules activities, everything. He doesn't have a clue about how to run a household."

Some women, like this student, clearly experience marriage as a stressor:

When we first started dating, I really loved him and thought he was wonderful. When I told him I didn't think I could be a medical student and his wife too, he said, "You're not going to give up your dream because of me." During the application process, he was very supportive. (Maybe he thought I wouldn't get in; I didn't think I would get in either.) Now, we're married, and I've discovered that being married while in medical school is damn near impossible. Among other things, he expects me to provide a full dinner every day from scratch. On the one hand, he wants a well-read wife, but on the other, he wants me home cooking and having babies. He picks fights just before exams and tells me, "I'm going to divorce you." Actually, I'd welcome a divorce, but if he leaves me what will I do? He pays one third of the rent and half the other bills.

You may be hard pressed to name any advantages to being the spouse of a medical student, but there are a few. "The fact that her husband is a medical student gives a wife some prestige among her coworkers," one student pointed out. "He can always take care of his wife if she gets sick, and their family can receive some of the best medical care in the area." Another added, "I think one compensation for a husband with a wife in medical school is not coming home to a dissatisfied spouse. I'm more interesting than when I stayed home with the children all day."

What are the disadvantages for a medical spouse?

It's a long, hard struggle from medical school through residency. The student's spouse is probably going to be the main breadwinner, and they're not going to be very well off financially. She won't see him very much, and when she does see him, he'll often be too tired or preoccupied with a patient or something. She might very likely feel she's playing second fiddle to medicine.

"I see very few advantages for a woman to be married to a physician except prestige and financial stability. I hope my wife doesn't feel this way!" If the wife is the medical student, her husband has to adjust to a nontraditional marriage. "Men who come from traditional families know that they will be waited on and cared for, have home-cooked meals—you just don't get that if you're married to a female medical student."

Because medical needs are usually considered more urgent than familial needs, absenteeism of the doctor from the home is common. Other sources of strain include the doctor's devaluing of the spouse as compared to work associates, the doctor's frustration of feeling less status and respect at home than at work; and the tendency to adopt an infallible clinical posture with family members (problems at home cannot be my fault, I'm the healer). Weakened by these strains, physicians' marriages too often evolve into "empty shell" relationships in which partners lead increasingly separate lives. Physicians' spouses often feel abandoned, depressed, and resentful, feelings exacerbated by guilt: "Here I am, feeling resentful because my doctor-spouse is out saving lives."

Marriage, like a garden, flourishes with care and attention. For your relationship to prosper, you must give some quality time.

The stress of school definitely exacts a toll on any relationship, no matter how stable it is. It's very important to make time for one's partner even if it means only one day a month where you devote all your time to the other person and not take him or her for granted.

"We keep our long-term goals in mind—we constantly tell each other that training will not last forever. Thus far our marriage has done wonderfully."

Division of Labor

Somebody has to wash the dishes. Many single men in medical school consider freedom from such "scut work" a major benefit of being married. In practice, of course, where one spouse is in medical school and the other is working outside the home or is in school, certain conflicts *can* arise over domestic duties. Some men sheepishly admit their tendency to leave these tasks to their wives. "She has to work, and she comes home worn out and then makes the meals and washes the dishes and does the laundry and takes care of practically all the bills and just runs the household while I'm booking it. Sometimes, it makes me feel uncomfortably guilty!" "When my wife comes home from work tired and I have a test the next day and can't give her any help, she gets irritated." "In the summer, I'm more willing to help around the house, but when school starts I don't do anything. I study and she works. I'm no help at all." "She's in school, too. When she has to work and I'm not too pushed, I wash dishes, clean up, and stuff. If I have work and she does, too, then we just let it go." "At times, my wife feels she is being used—that she's just there to do the washing and cooking."

And female medical students are frustrated by traditional expectations. "Intellectually, we know we have to share the workload, but when it comes down to the fact the laundry hasn't been done for two weeks, I'm the one who's going to do it." "My being in medical school hasn't affected our division of labor, except maybe to the extent that my husband now takes our children to the doctor and dentist." "Women medical students still feel social expectations (even if they have liberal mates); the conflict between role expectations in medical school and role expectations at home can put women in a precarious situation." "Marriage and medical school would be more compatible if I could hire a maid!" As one female physician noted, "Clearly, medicine was set up and developed for men, not women."

Other couples take a more equitable, if necessarily casual, approach to domestic chores. "We both hated housework, so we always did it together. We use it as a study break—study for an hour and then do the dishes. And while cleaning the dishes we'll talk, bitch, and discuss our goals. It makes the chores more bearable." "My husband and I are both in school and very busy. The only way we get by is to let the mess build up and not get stressed by it. Eventually, one of us will get some free time to clean things up."

Decision making can be authoritarian. "One of us has to give in and it's usually my wife," said a physician-in-training with domineering tendencies. "On a long-term basis, what can you do?" Others are more egalitarian. "When we come to a disagreement we can't resolve by compromise, the decision depends on who'd be most affected. That one has the final say."

Leisure Time

Married or single, medical students devote enormous amounts of time to study and, in later years, to their clinical practice. Sometimes, the impact on a marriage is devastating. "Those 80-100 hour weeks didn't allow me to have a happy family. The time strains placed on our relationship caused a domino effect that lead to our divorce. Eight years down the drain!" Work pressures can be a major cause of strife and disappointment. "It's tough on my wife when she works hard all week not to do anything on the weekend, but I've got to study." "My wife and I have always tried to go out on Saturday night, even just to a movie. There have been an awful lot of times in the past two months when we didn't go anywhere for fun."

> Every hour I spend with my wife is an hour I could have been studying. I finally admitted to myself it would have been a lot easier the first year if we hadn't been married—I could have just gone off for a couple months and got the studying done. It would have prevented a lot of problems.

"This weekend we planned on going to a movie, so I started calling around for a baby-sitter. Only, I didn't know any baby-sitters. That bothered me."

This student expressed the frustrations of medical students married to each other:

> All I know is that she can't be there for me and I can't be there for her either. I needed to understand that she wasn't rejecting me on a personal level—she was spending so much time in the hospital. I knew it in my head, but until we talked it out I still felt miserable. We decided to read together several times a week and to go out on a date at least once a week.

Some couples comfortably accommodate to the hectic schedule and even see benefits to their limited time together. "I appreciate my wife more than I did when I could be with her all the time," one student said. "I think what counts is the quality, not the quantity, of time you spend with your family."

But there is a problem with this philosophy, as this female student notes: "You get into trouble if you set aside time for your mate/family with the expectation that it's going to be dynamite. Usually the good times arise fairly spontaneously and you have to be around long enough to let them emerge. They can't really be scheduled." Along the same lines, another student explains, "I used to tell myself, 'We're going to have fantastic fun tonight.' Then, I would be depressed all evening because I wasn't having all that much fun."

The pressure of exams and deadlines can stifle romance. And for some newlyweds who had little time to become really well acquainted before training began, it can be particularly harrowing. "We got married five days before medical school started and had some problems adjusting to one another."

> It's bad studying every night and then your wife has to work and comes home from work with her problems. It sort of limits you to weekends. If you're studying on weekends for a quiz, it really messes things up— makes sexual relations sort of a hit-and-miss thing. I'm geared for more sexual activity, but either I'm too busy or my wife's too busy. It gets on your nerves.

Deferred sexuality, a problem for unmarried students, also afflicts the married. "Even though I'm married, medical school affects my sex life before exams. Sometimes, I don't even have a sex drive because I'm so preoccupied." "I'm up an awful lot when she's asleep. We go to bed together maybe once a week at best." Women students, too, express frustration. "I usually go to bed about two o'clock, and he goes to bed about midnight so . . . "

> Sex got to be a joke. We would both be so keyed up and stressed out that it wouldn't be any fun. My married girlfriend and I would call each other up to report a good sexual encounter, usually once every few weeks. You start to worry that you and your spouse aren't normal, that there must be something wrong with only having sex once or twice a month. But if you consider the stress you're under, it's really a normal response. If you're both not bothered by it, then enjoy it when you can!

Children

When to start a family often puzzles married students. "I always expected that when you get married you have children; that's the way it is—the natural progression of things. I was devastated when my wife told me we couldn't have children while she was in medical training." Yet, he could see her point of view: "It's irrational for me to marry a medical student and then expect to have children right away. She can't quit school or take time off, so I've had to revise my timeline."

Having children can seriously impact the already precarious economic status of a couple. "We've been married five years," one student said, "and we'd really love to have a kid right now, but financially there's no way." On the other hand, some couples are reluctant to wait until completion of training to begin a family.

The difficulty of the decision is compounded for female students. Parenthood and medicine are both so time consuming that many women devote themselves entirely to the former and many men entirely to the latter. A female medical student and mother must make major compromises at work, at home, or both. "Whether she is a medical student or not," one pointed out, "a woman has the responsibility for the kids. Men have it a lot easier." Despite these problems, they are envied by some women. "I'm single and I worry about when will there be time to get married and to have kids? I'm envious of those who are already married. They're ahead of the game."

Should a woman student take time off from school or continue on, missing those early experiences of being a mom? Many female students are opting to go ahead and have children. An AAMC report notes that 11% of female medical graduates reported one or more dependents.[2] "If I were to take a year off later on between my fourth year and internship, then my child would be a year old, and I'd never see it while in my residency. But if I wait until I finish, I'd be getting pretty old."

Both married and single parents in medical school have trouble finding sufficient time and energy for parenting. "The absolute minimum that I will spend with my son is one day a week. That doesn't sound like much, but the way the system is, they expect you to be nothing but a student." And for a student mother, there are considerable difficulties in finding, keeping, and financing adequate child care.

Medical students increasingly question the necessity of the physician as absentee spouse and parent. Some wonder if it's really necessary for a dedicated physician to sacrifice family life on the altar of medicine.

Just because your training requires 80 hours a week or more doesn't mean you have to keep up that grueling pace for the rest of your life. A surgeon sat a group of us third-year students down one day and said: "Decide what problem in the world you would like to solve and go for it." That was okay. But then he said, "The reason you are working 100-plus hours a week is because you are driven. Don't think it will end when you are out of training, because it won't. You will keep up that same pace, because you love it." Well, later we found out that this man's wife had divorced him, he never spent time with his two children, and he was very unhappy in his personal life. These are not the kind of role models we need, but they are often the only ones available to us.

Marriage can be a great learning and growing experience for both part-ners. "If I had it to do over again," a graduating senior said, "I would get married and go to school. What I have learned by working through our marital problems has helped me become a more compassionate person. It will help me in the long run with my patients."

Your challenge as an emerging physician is to develop a balanced per-spective and lifestyle. Taking the necessary time out to keep your important relationships vital will enhance, not diminish, your health, well-being, and professional career.

Insights: Healthy Relationships
Bernard Virshup, MD

A healthy relationship is an important resource in coping with stress and counteracting the debilitating isolation that can occur while pursuing a medi-cal career. But good relationships are the result of knowledgeable and even sophisticated behaviors. Many medical students are socially unsophisticated. Many are likely to be introverts who are willing to spend a lot of time alone and who interact infrequently and less successfully with others. They are apt to think more of their own needs than those of their partner and to be more concerned with their needs being met than meeting those of their partner. This can be a very big mistake, ending in neither getting their needs met.

Those with a relationship with someone in medicine have two major and very serious complaints. The first is that there is so little time spent together. Although medicine is demanding, you must, if you are to have a successful relationship, allocate enough time to it. It need not be as much time as either of you would like, but it must be enough time. You cannot let other consid-erations get in the way.

A second complaint is that when a couple is together, the medical student (or physician) won't talk about feelings, the relationship, or problems. This does not make for a healthy relationship. What is a healthy relationship? These qualities seem important:

Empathy: I can see the world through the eyes of the other person. I understand because I can get inside the other's skin. I listen well to all the cues, both verbal and nonverbal, that the other person sends, and I respond to these cues.

Feelings and emotions: I'm not afraid to deal directly with emotions, my own or the other's. I allow myself both to feel and to give expression in my relationship to what I feel. I expect my partner to do the same, but I do not inflict my emotions on him or her.

Genuineness: I am genuine rather than phony when interacting. I don't hide behind roles or facades; my partner knows where I stand.

Self-disclosure: I let my partner see the person inside; I use self-disclosure to help establish a sound relationship with him or her.

Admiration and respect: I feel and demonstrate admiration and respect for my partner as a person of quality. I accept my partner even when I do not necessarily agree with or approve of what he or she does. I am an actively supportive person.

Commitment to each other's welfare and happiness: Commitment is the major binding force in a relationship—in spite of storms, reservations, hurt, anger, or fear of emotional closeness.

Basic trust: I know and trust that my partner has my best interests at heart, would not intentionally hurt me, and will be available when needed—in spite of inadvertent actions and comments that wound me because of prior experiences.

Initiative: In my relationship, I act rather than just react. I am spontaneous. I take the initiative. I am not passive.

Loyalty: I am an ally, not a judge. I will never embarrass, criticize, or correct my mate publicly.

In the courtship and honeymoon periods, we are apt to endow our partner with attributes they don't really have, attributes that we *wish* they had. That is, we "project" our inner needs and desires onto our partners, and they on us, and bask in the glow of our mutual admiration. Inevitably, reality emerges.

When someone fails to live up to our expectations in nonintimate relationships, we may feel disappointed, but adjust our expectations. We lower our expectations and bring them more into line with reality. In an intimate relationship, however, the response is frequently different: Failed expectations lead to hurt and anger, not necessarily a lowering of expectations. Each partner may regard the other's desires as signs of self-centeredness. The partners may then come to judge the other (but not themselves) as selfish, pig-headed, stingy, contrary, arbitrary, dumb, and childish.

When, after the first flush of intimacy, our expectations of another are met with disappointment, we have a choice: Either the other person is untrustworthy and a scumbag—we made a terrible mistake trusting him or her—or our expectations were unrealistic and we should adjust them to reality. We almost always decide the first. The second is almost invariably true. We all begin with expectations that people who care about us will be sensitive to our needs and giving. We find with dismay that even people who care about us must take care of their own needs first.

We think, why should I be the one to change? There's nothing wrong with me. The problem is my partner. If my partner would shape up, everything would be fine. I won't make an effort unless my partner does. It's not fair for me to have to do all the work.

The truth is, that it is we and our unrealistic expectations that must change so we can appreciate the remarkable person who has come into our life. It is much more important to discover how another person *is* than whether or not he or she meets our adolescent fantasies. If you encourage your partner to be and become the unique, valuable person he or she is capable of being, rather than a mere appendage to your career, it is you who will reap the benefits.

The following are some of the unrealistic expectations and beliefs that almost always lead to a troubled relationship: My partner

- will, above all, respect my career, identify with it, share it with me, and support my efforts
- will be available for sex whenever I want (need) it, for this is evidence of love
- will do what I want without being asked
- will do the household chores and have dinner ready for me
- will understand and be forgiving when, tired and impatient, I snap at him or her
- will take care of me
- will know when I am feeling bad or need help and behave supportively
- will shape his or her life to fit mine
- will not do anything he or she knows I can't stand
- will not quarrel with me if he or she truly loves me

And finally, "I deserve to be happy. It's unfair that life is so difficult."

When unrealistic expectations meet reality we are, for a while, confused, depressed, and angry. But when we readjust our expectations to reality, we discover that reality and growing up are rather nice.[3,4]

Notes

1. Coombs, R. H., and Faway I. Fawzy. 1982, November. "The Effect of Marital Status on Stress in Medical School." *American Journal of Psychiatry,* 139(11):1490-1493.

2. Wiebe, Christine. 1995, March. "From Here to Maternity." *The New Physician,* pp. 41-44.

3. Truax, Charles B., and Robert R. Carkhuff. 1967. *Toward Effective Counseling and Psychotherapy: Training, Practice.* Chicago: Aldine.

4. Beck, Aaron T. 1988. *Love Is Never Enough: How Couples Can Overcome Misunderstandings, Resolve Conflicts, and Solve Relationship Problems Through Cognitive Therapy.* New York: Harper & Row.

CHAPTER 6

Third Year

Who's the Real Doc Here?

The third year is mainly a feeling of walking around not knowing what you're doing.

—Third-year medical student

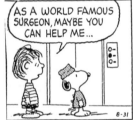
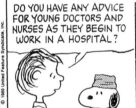
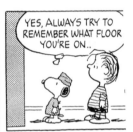

As a third-year student, you get your long-awaited opportunity to function almost to full capacity as part of a clinical team—and you may find yourself frighteningly unprepared for the experience. It is rare for a student to feel totally confident going in, and these feelings are intensified by hospital staff who ask, "Haven't you learned that yet?"

Patients rarely present themselves as textbook examples. Procedures that sounded simple and logical on paper are confusing in the hospital room. Gone are the days when you could do well simply by studying textbooks and lecture notes. No longer will the most effective way to start an IV on a child come to you recipe-style from a book. You will organize and integrate important information learned from seriously ill and occasionally hostile patients who have already been interviewed two or three times by a variety of hospital personnel. Everyone else around you will seem busily functioning and ministering to patients while you aren't even sure how to stay out of the way.

The third year is divided into clerkships. You and your classmates will randomly rotate through internal medicine, surgery, ob/gyn, pediatrics, neurology, psychiatry, and so on. Each specialty has its own routine, rules of conduct, and organizational idiosyncracies. You may feel like a traveler in a foreign country. How late is the cafeteria open? Where are the chest films kept after 5 p.m.? What is the phone number of the patient escort service? Where can family members wait while I do physical exams? How was I supposed to know that they don't do endoscopies on Friday?

> There is an amazing transition when the clinical work begins. For years—before and during medical school and on the boards—you've been conditioned to learn lots and lots of facts, and the major factor in your measured worth is how much you know—mostly on multiple choice tests. (Multiple choice! Where I went to college, these were considered inferior instruments that required no real knowledge!) Suddenly, abruptly, when you begin to work on the wards, and presumably for the rest of your working life, the emphasis changes. You are still expected to know things, as well as to learn more; you get pimped [put in my place] and live in fear of not knowing the appropriate fact of the moment; but all of a sudden, the truly most important thing about you is no longer your information but your ethics, believe it or not. All sorts of stuff you need to have learned from your mother becomes critical. You need to be reliable, diligent, honest, interested, respectful, and easy to work with. You will be *evaluated* on these characteristics on the same level as for your "knowledge base." So, for the basic science drudge who doubts he'll ever be able to know enough, take heart. You actually get credits for being a decent person.

Clinical Assignment

Typically, the transition from basic science student to apprentice clinician feels abrupt, unsettling, and not as you anticipated. "I felt helplessly lost and I didn't think I'd ever catch on," said a third-year medical student. Some teaching hospitals formally structure an orientation to the clinical floors to make it less threatening. At other hospitals, students are given a self-help orientation manual with hand-me-down tips from the previous class titled

something like "How To Survive the Clinical Years." So, although some dis-
orientation is inevitable, some students make the transition with relative ease.
They may have prepared themselves during the first two years by following
preceptors engaged in clinical activities, by taking part in summer externship
programs, or by finding temporary or part-time employment in a hospital or
clinic. "For me, this year wasn't much of a problem. I had tremendous instruction the summer prior to my clerkships, so it was a real relaxed situation."

Whether it happens during the final weeks of your sophomore year or
thereafter, you will probably experience at least a few confusing days when
you feel thrown out on the floors for the first time and lost in another world.
Each time you rotate onto a new service, you will be forced to adapt quickly
and unobtrusively to a new routine. "The first three days, I didn't get home
until after midnight. I had visions that this was what medicine would be like
for the rest of my life, and I knew I couldn't handle the pace." "It took me
hours to do things I now do in five or ten minutes. Starting an IV seemed like
doing neurosurgery. Everything was a big deal back then." "Besides dealing
with patients for the first time, you have to keep asking people where everything is kept, and they're busy and don't want to keep answering your questions. You can start off on the wrong foot." "Just when you start to catch on,
you're thrown into a new situation with new people, new problems, new patients, and new locations. It's back to square one."

But when the confusion abates and once-difficult tasks become routine,
you'll probably agree, "I feel pretty good about it." "I'm happy to finally be
out of the classroom and doing the clinical work I've looked forward to for
so many years." "It's a really good feeling," a classmate added, "Another
milestone passed."

Responsibilities

Depending on the service and the hospital, you may be expected to "do
as little as you can" and essentially stay out of the way and watch: "Say the
least, get along the best." On some services, students feel they receive little
or no actual teaching, and what they learn they acquire on their own. "You're
sort of lost, really. There's no orientation on surgery. There was some on
medicine, but by the time I got there I already knew all I'd need to know about
the floor." "Sometimes, you're ignored. You ask a question and it's like no one
hears you." "In pediatrics and ob/gyn, they've taken the trouble to teach us,
but in the subspecialties they haven't. Maybe, we're just in the way. If I were
a neurosurgical or orthopedic resident, I wouldn't ask a medical student to do

procedures. The residents are there to learn, too, but they're doing things we could be doing."

On another service or at another hospital, the opposite may be true. "They keep you so busy you don't have time to read up on a patient even if you wanted to." "Sometimes you feel you have more than you can handle. Before, it was mental exhaustion, now it's just physical." The workload can over-whelm a newcomer, even on a relatively slow service, because "Everything takes so long when you're unaccustomed to taking histories, doing work-ups, filling out orders and reports, and completing third-year-type write-ups" and because the general routine is unfamiliar and mystifying. This is how one third-year student remembers his first minutes in the ER:

A loudspeaker above the triage station blares: "16-year-old boy, gunshot wound to the abdomen, vitals stable, ETA three minutes." I freeze for a second. A resident throws me a gown and cries, "Put that on! The masks are over there. Draw the ABG and insert the Foley when he comes in." I take a deep breath and think to myself, "This is it. Am I ready?"[1]

Some residents, and even some nurses, expect medical students to do a substantial amount of scut work, much of it of the 3 a.m. variety. "Anybody who can keeps passing routine tasks along until they get down to the third-year student." "The third-year students wind up doing most of the scut work, but I guess we have to learn how to do some of that stuff, too." "Residents take a bit of advantage, calling you late at night to start an IV. It might take you half an hour to get to the hospital and do it—something he or she could do in five or ten minutes—but for whatever reason, the call comes."

As a third- and fourth-year student, you'll be expected to be much more thorough in your history taking and write-ups than the interns and residents. Much more thorough, in fact, than you'll want to be. Some third-year students report spending as much as three to four hours on a single physical examination. Much of it is spent in checking and rechecking against "cue cards" to make sure nothing has been omitted and trying to make sure you remember what the patient said. This need to refer constantly to notes can damage an already tender self-image. "I had an absolute horror of going in to see patients because I knew I had to read my cue cards in order to work them up. It was really embarrassing." "Sometimes I'd wonder, 'How long should I listen to this guy's heart? I really don't know what I'm hearing and if I listen too long, he'll know I don't know what I'm doing, or worse yet, he might start worrying that I've found something wrong with his heart.'"

And it's so embarrassing to walk back into a patient's room to ask another question or do another part of the exam you forgot. Sometimes, you're so overwhelmed by getting everything that you forget to focus. You may see a patient with abdominal pain and think you did a thorough H&P [history and physical] only to have the attending ask about what food the patient ate previously. You feel stupid saying, "Oh, I forgot to ask."

Gradually, you'll become more comfortable about your diagnostic acumen. You'll actually begin performing hands-on procedures—drawing blood, doing heel sticks on infants, starting IVs, doing lumbar punctures—in a fairly routine manner. "The first time I had to do a bone marrow, I couldn't think about anything else for three hours before. I was conscious of how the patient felt, scared to death I'd hurt him. But when you've done a few, you can put that aside and figure what you're doing is for his benefit."

You'll discover heavy demands are paired with limited actual responsibilities. For example, you cannot sign orders or prescribe, although you may be expected to write the orders and ask an MD to cosign them. As you become more comfortable with your duties, you'll probably begin to feel frustrated with these limitations. "I feel like a glorified secretary when I go up to a resident with five things for her to sign." "I wish we had more responsibility for patient care. I feel like I'm not doing a damn thing." "I've been doing academic work a long time, and when I finally got on the floor I felt really excited. But our diagnoses aren't even looked at."

You'll be expected to suggest courses of treatment and medications and to interact closely with patients on your service—listening, explaining, answering questions when possible, and generally learning "bedside manner." In fact, because interns and residents are so overloaded, you'll often find yourself the "doctor" with the greatest opportunity to spend time with patients. "Actually, this can be the most rewarding time in your career, with minimal responsibility and maximum satisfaction."

Students enjoy the realization that they can play an important role with patients. "I found I could influence a patient's emotional status by my mood."

Especially on the service floors where they don't have regular doctors, the patients don't get real close attention, and the third-year student is the one who can spend the most time with them and explain things. They really appreciate it when you take time to stop by and just shoot the breeze.

In other situations, there may not be much time for this. "Chatting pleasantly with patients is not encouraged and is indirectly discouraged through assignments that keep you too busy." And accessibility can create repercussions:

A lot of the time, other members of the team are so pressured that the family of a patient who is chronically ill or going down fast looks to the third-year student to explain what's going on. I've gotten cornered a couple of times and that can get to you pretty fast.

"It's okay to say, 'I don't know, but I'll get someone who does to go over that with you.'" "You have to know what topics to leave up to the attending physician—like serious diagnoses or complications resulting from procedures." This student, however, one month into his clinical training, was the only one available when a patient died:

His son came into the team room, where I sat alone, and said to me in a shaky voice, "I think my dad's stopped breathing." With no one else around, not knowing what else to do, I ran into the room and placed my stethoscope on his quiet chest, straining to hear some sound. I wanted him just to be kidding, to wake up laughing and shouting, "I had you fooled!" Instead he was silent. His son and daughter-in-law looked at me with the wide eyes of terror and knowledge. They knew the reality but wanted so desperately to hear some other news. . . . I mustered the artificial confidence shared by every M-3 and told a young man that his father had died. I told him as gently as I could, with empathy and compassion.[2]

These and other encounters dictate learning experiences. "There's a big change in how you learn. There's no assigned reading; instead, it's up to you to find relevant material to read. There are fewer tests. Much of your learning is self-motivated during the clinical years."

With the onset of clinical responsibilities, the medical student often gets a first taste of the workload notorious among interns and residents. As a third-year student, Adriane Fugh-Berman held this conversation with a nonmedical student:

"What a great rotation!" I said to a Regular Person. "We don't have to be in till seven [a.m.] and we're usually out by seven at night, unless we're on call. And we don't have to work every weekend!" My friend gave me one of those get-the-straitjacket looks and said, "You're happy about only working twelve hours a day?" "Well, yeah," I said, surprised.

On another occasion, her nonmedical friend couldn't understand why she couldn't take time off for a special event:

"You must see the Matisse exhibit, but go on a weekday, it's less crowded." "Elana, I can't do anything on the weekday, and rarely on the weekend," I said. "We're in the hospital all the time now." Elana gave me a haughty and uncomprehending look. "But this is a once in a lifetime opportunity," she said. "Tell them that it's very important for you to go." I felt like I was looking at Elana from the bottom of a well. How to explain the complete lack of control that one has over one's life in third year. Maybe I should tell her the story of what I had to go through to get out of three hours of surgery when I had been subpoenaed by a Federal court. "Tell them you're a doctor and you can't go, my resident told me."[3]

Hospital Personnel

Students who might forget their neophyte status on the wards are usually quickly reminded. They are at the bottom of the medical pecking order and are expected to behave accordingly. Usually a third-year student cannot work up a patient before that patient has been seen by a fourth-year student, an intern, or a resident. So, the third-year student is frequently the third or fourth person to go over the same ground and perform the same physical examinations and may consequently become the target of the patient's annoyance.

Students must be on hand for rounds and conferences and are not permitted to make excuses—such as classes they should be attending—when a senior medical officer decides an informal lecture is in order. "There are many conflicts of time and responsibility. You are expected to attend student conferences, take care of your patients, read on your own, meet with attendings, go on rounds, etc. These are often mutually exclusive and it is hard to know what to do."

The attending physician is typically the most powerful figure in the hospital hierarchy—a hierarchy ranging on down in order through various residents, interns, and nurses. This is how one student describes the attending physician:

Also known as "the attending" or, in some cases, "The Attending!". . . This is the person with ultimate responsibility for the care of patients. All major decisions about patient management are cleared by the attending. . . . In general, it is probably prudent to run questions and therapeutic suggestions by the residents before presenting them to the attendings. And it would be a grave political error to present a significant finding or lab result during attending rounds without presenting that information to the residents first.[4]

As mentioned, third-year students may often face "pimping" by attending physicians and residents. Although the alleged purpose of pimping is to test knowledge or teach, it often illuminates the third-year student's lowly status and shaky confidence. Eric Whitaker writes of such an experience:

As a freshly minted third year student I reported to the surgical floors, ready to impress. The chief resident asked that I learn everything there was to know about breast cancer to present the following day. After much study, the moment of truth arrived—morning rounds. As I readied to blurt out the epidemiology and pathophysiology of breast cancer, the chief resident shifted gears. He began to rifle me with questions about reggae groups from the 1960s and before. I knew very little about reggae groups that predated my birth and so performed poorly. The resident made the point that there would always be something I did not know and he would find it. And he did it before a group of my peers. I brushed the mental assault aside until I recounted the incident to my dean. She was angered. The chief resident's questions did not contribute to my education or patient care, she said. Further, the cumulative effects of such minor episodes contribute to increased stress in an already stressful environment.[5]

Although not all attending physicians or residents take their authority to such an extreme, grilling medical students is a fairly common practice. Fortunately, many residents are knowledgeable and willing to answer students' questions without humiliating them.

Most interns—PGY-1 (postgraduate year 1)—tend to be patient and fair, still remembering vividly what it was like to be a med student. "They're closest to us and the easiest doctors to talk to," one said. "They're pretty unsure of themselves, too, I think, so they're easier to approach." A few, however, are smitten with their new status and try to distance themselves from lowly students. "They stand just a little bit taller," one student said "and discourage students from showing too much familiarity." "It's 'Doctor' to you," another student said. Such an attitude, though, is atypical. Residents, although not unkind, generally have little time or patience for listening to or answering student questions. This is both understandable and annoying. "They have the most patient responsibility and the least time for students," one explained. "A few of them tend to look on us as excess baggage." "It really depends on which services you are on. Some residents are untouchable. But others regard it their duty to teach students and do a good job of it." "If a resident is good and teaches you, students work hard and may stay way past what is necessary. But if the resident is a 'jerk' or too stressed out, students will just 'disappear.'"

Relationships with the nursing staff can also be tricky. Some nursing supervisors specify that there will be "no fraternizing" between students and nurses and emphasize that the relationship should be kept on a "Dr. So-and-so" and "Nurse So-and-so" basis. Some nurses themselves make that rule abundantly clear.

In other settings, however, medical students, nurses, and residents work comfortably on a first-name basis. Sometimes, nurses may seem overly familiar. Seniors may advise you to intern elsewhere to escape nurses you've "grown up with." Otherwise you'll *always* be treated as students, especially by older nurses who consider you "their little boys and girls."

Women students occasionally complain about the chumminess some female nurses display toward them, in contrast to the "obsequiousness they may show toward the male house staff." Conversely, other women students are surprised when nurses are not friendlier toward them. "I thought I would get along easily with the nurses in a friendly, personal way, but I was surprised to be treated as a 'Doctor' in a polite and cooperative way."

Those students who readily admit their confusion and uncertainty in the unfamiliar hospital environment and who acknowledge and show respect for nurses generally find them helpful and willing to go out of their way to keep them from making dangerous errors. "They realize you've just started, and they try to help by being courteous and not belittling you. They're my favorite people."

Students who feel they must keep the upper hand with nurses often meet with disastrous results. "I chewed out a nurse for keeping me waiting 45 minutes and being lazy—*never* do this as a student!—and for three days the nurses wouldn't help me. They even asked me to change a sheet when I got blood on it." "If you give a nurse a hard time, they all hear about it and you can see their attitudes change. Cross them and they'll make life miserable." "A word to the wise," one student warned, "grow up and work together!"

Older nurses who have spent many years on hospital duty may be impatient with students who cause extra work without making any real contribution to patient care. Student nurses, on the other hand, play an important role in building up med student egos, not only because of their youth and their lowly status as fellow novices, but also because they tend to ask questions and to be impressed with the students' knowledge. They offer the best opportunity for third-year students to practice the time-honored medical dictum, "See one, do one, teach one."

One observant third-year student notes a paradoxical phenomenon among his peers:

> I am struck by a sense of frenzied self-absorption that permeates all our lives. Delivered from the classroom to the operating room, I realized one day that I was living with a new set of clothes, a new bewildering set of personal interactions, and apprehension of a physician's responsibility. In fewer than six months, I have invaded vessels with needles and catheters; I have seen craniotomies and open-heart surgery; I have performed CPR and open-heart massage during real code blue resuscitations; I've almost been mauled by a young woman with schizophrenia and spent hours talking to another woman suffering from profound, suicidal depression. I have witnessed so much. Now that I am immersed in doctoring, I've discovered new motivations for learning; yet, unfortunately, there is little time to read. Due to the time constraints and energy drain of third year, I lack the drive to assimilate any of these experiences.

Patients

The degree of patient contact third-year students experience varies from hospital to hospital and from service to service. Some students deplore minimal contact, feeling "We don't see all the things we want to." The fewer patients seen, the slower the learning process. "You have to be around a lot of patients and see a lot of things before you really remember."

On the other hand, students with a light patient load get better acquainted with patients and can spend time in the library reading about their conditions.

And, of course, the students' notions of what constitutes a heavy patient load varies with their own experience and competence. "At first, I didn't want to see many patients because it was too traumatic. If I had one patient to work up in a day, it was slavery! As I became more self-assured, I wanted to see more. As time passes, you learn to work faster."

You may find yourself complaining about too few patients one day and too many the next. "Sometimes, I think I'd like to see more patients; but then at other times I wish I were alone in a corner." On most services, the schedule is "Hurry up and wait," because you can't program people's illnesses. "It comes in spurts. Sometimes, you have a whole bunch and no time to learn about them, and then you'll only have a couple." "On Ob, you like patients to come in when you have nothing to do. But usually they come in after you've gone to bed." "It's worse being bored and stuck in a hospital. If I have to be there all day, let me work!"

At a large medical center, your experience may be with specialized cases referred from other hospitals. "We haven't seen much 'bread and butter' medicine, mostly a lot of exotic stuff." This emphasis on the unusual reinforces a tendency to "not look for the common thing. What pops into my mind is some strange syndrome they mentioned in pathology. I don't remember what's common, because they didn't stress that." "Like they say, 'When I hear hoofbeats, I tend to look for zebras, not horses.'"

How you'll react to the patients you see will depend to a great extent on your own—and your patients'—personality and perhaps on your gender, socioeconomic background, and age. Initially, your reactions will likely be colored by insecurity: "I have a lot of trouble knowing how to approach patients. I feel funny. I'm not a doctor, but I have to walk in there and 'play' doctor."

If you're a woman, you may find yourself, as one said, "more into the personal, sympathetic attitude. Men tend to move right into the clinical aspect with a lot of technical questions. That's their pattern of reaction." A woman explained, "When I'm evaluated by men, I'm always told that I sometimes get too involved with my patients. I don't believe my patients ever think so, and I don't really think it's wrong." Another woman adds, "Other doctors recognize patients' emotional problems, but they respond on an intellectual level. I respond emotionally, but I don't think I let patients see it."

In an era when physicians are increasingly coming under fire for an emotionally sterile approach to patient care, the tendency of many women to be openly nurturing and responsive to their patients may have a beneficial effect on their male counterparts. Legitimizing expressions of feelings, suppressed in the traditional macho approach to patient relations, adds a humanistic depth to patient care.

Students of both sexes see themselves as more sensitive to patients' feelings than older clinicians are. Consider the evident dismay of this medical student assigned to observe labor and delivery:

> Along with two other medical students, I reported to the chief resident and then loitered in the hallway, listening for several hours. Finally, we were alerted that someone's delivery was imminent. . . . Seven people now attended her delivery. As the woman stared at us between wrenching contractions, the chief resident explained that we were medical students. She did not solicit the patient's consent, but chirped, "This is the first birth they've ever seen, so let's put on a good show for them, okay?"[6]

"One insensitive doctor told us that all medical students our age are concerned about patients' feelings because we don't know anything yet. Once we learn what's involved in taking care of patients, he said, your feelings will go out the window. I hope that isn't true!"

Patients' Attitudes

Students find acceptance by patients astonishing. "Surprisingly, they consider us their doctors!" "Some of them really seem to believe what I tell them and accept it at face value." "And they answer any question!" Indigent patients are often less perceptive than private patients of the subtler distinctions in the medical hierarchy and just assume "Everybody's a doctor, some doctors are just younger than others." By contrast, private patients, expecting to be attended by their personal physicians, can be more difficult. They resent interrogation or being "practiced on" by students and want "only professional people around them." Fortunately, some attending physicians explain to them that the teaching role is an important function in any medical center. Others leave it to the students to work it out with patients as best they can.

Typically, it's up to the individual student to decide whether to explain his or her actual rank. Some are scrupulous about identifying their student role, whereas others prefer not to raise the subject. "How to introduce yourself is always a big concern. Should it be 'student doctor,' 'medical student,' or just my first name?" Being explicit about student status can save later embarrassment. Since you may know very little about the resident's plans for a particular patient—even if you do understand the facts of the case—you will be routinely placed in the position of answering, "I don't know," or "Why don't you discuss that with your resident?" It's easier to be frank than to mislead or misinform an inquiring patient or reveal information that should be left to the resident. "Be honest!" one student advises. "Lying will get you nowhere, and patients can tell anyway by your position in the pack." "Don't cover your name tag or stop wearing it. Be proud that you're learning to be the best physician possible." "Typically, I'll introduce myself by saying, 'Hi, I'm so-and-so, a member of the medical team taking care of you while you're here.' If they ask, I always say I'm a student physician."

Some patients, recognizing that they are dealing with a student, adopt the mentor role and explain their symptoms, discuss their cases, and otherwise "help teach." Although you may appreciate patients who are "tolerant and allow you to do procedures that are repeated for your benefit," you may become skeptical of excessive cooperation. Over-enthusiasm, the mark of a "professional patient," is characteristic of patients who, although they may have a genuine ailment, thoroughly enjoy the attention afforded by the sick role. For them, being a patient is a way of life, a revolving-door existence in and out of clinics. Since the information these patients convey may be inflated or otherwise inaccurate or irrelevant, they can "waste time" and become the antithesis of "efficient medicine":

> We get a lot of professional patients in the clinic who get a kick out of being diagnosed. They're either 'showboats' or just extremely interested in helping you to learn, but some of them carry on, build a whole big story, throw in a few jokes—it's like a nightclub routine.

Patients can also unnerve student doctors. "A few of the older patients remarked on how young I am. One lady I examined told me, 'You're too young to be doing this.'" Occasionally, patients may not cooperate:

> On my psych rotation, I was in the ER and this male patient refused to talk to me. When the resident came out and asked what was wrong, the patient said he couldn't talk to me because I was a woman, and an attractive woman at that. I just stood there totally in limbo not knowing what to say. Fortunately, my resident looked at the patient and said, "Look, she's here to talk to you and knows what to do; if you don't like it, leave!" The patient ended up talking to me.

For some patients, being the object lesson in medical pathology and care is discomforting. "It's so hard to see a patient just to see a rash or something, not to care for the patient. I feel like I'm invading someone's privacy. What do you say to a patient? 'Hi, I'm here to see your disease?'" One woman objected to the "number of people traipsing in and out of patients' rooms here." An attending physician, several residents, and a number of medical students had entered her room to examine the woman in the bed next to hers. The "retinue," she protested, "was all male. There was not even a token female." The medical students "all carried notebooks," in which they busily wrote, heads down, while the attending spoke at the bedside. "They referred to this woman in the third person throughout" and "turned their backs on her several times. It was utterly dehumanizing."[7]

The former national poet laureate Josephine Jacobson described teaching rounds during her hospital stay metaphorically "as 'Dr. Logan and his crew board[ing] the ship of her room.' . . . Now the immaculate figures gathered around her bed, as though she were an unexpected golden egg laid by a provident goose during the night."[8]

Students' Views of Patients

Although you will have little choice regarding the patients you treat, you will develop opinions concerning good and bad ones. Aside from those who are very ill and with whom direct interaction is consequently limited, patients seem to fall into categories. Most are "pretty nice" and cooperative, but some are "real hard on you, abusive, won't subject themselves to treatment or accept medication; they're tough for a medical student to work with." You will no doubt quickly learn to spot both the "professional patients" and the "crocks"—those whose complaints have (or seem to have) no organic origin. Some students use slang terms whereas others, like this student, reject them as offensive: "These terms are used in an extremely derogatory manner and I think they're terrible!"

The distinction between "good" and "bad" patients typically relates to their personalities and the quality of your relationship with them. "A good patient is one who communicates and who understands the physician's questions and instructions." "Good patients follow what you ask them to do. They're smart enough to understand what the problem is, can accept that they're sick and need treatment, and are intelligent enough to ask questions and understand the answers." "Good patients are interested in getting themselves well." "A good patient is appreciative."

A "bad or difficult patient is one who will not follow orders and doesn't want to get well." They wait too long to come in for treatment, thereby making it harder for their physicians to effectively treat them. "Bad" patients also "fight you every step of the way" and "constantly doubt what you say." One student noted, however, that "Many patients who fight you seem to recover very well. Maybe they fight their disease as vigorously as they fight you!" One of my most humanistic attendings reminded us, "No matter what's happening to you, the patient is always having a worse day."

"Crocks," difficult patients whose many complaints have no discoverable organic cause, are also "bad" patients. Because they have emotional problems behind their physical complaints, residents "dump them" on students: "Residents give them to us because they are tired of seeing them."

Students are sometimes overwhelmed by such patients. "If I see too many of them, I'm going to wind up missing something pretty soon because I'll be too quick to label somebody a crock who isn't." Indeed, a patient who has all the signs of being a genuine crock may suddenly manifest acute physical symptoms, providing a frightening and very instructive lesson about ailments that are thought to be "all in the head."

Some students are uncomfortable treating children because they must deal with parents. "What really bothers me is examining the patient with the mother standing over me." "You have to take care of the child, the father, the mother, sometimes the grandmother and brothers and sisters, especially if you deal with chronic illness or some psychological problem." And, as many parents would agree, "Little kids are hard to handle—uncooperative." On the other hand, you will discover compensating factors in dealing with children: "They're sick, and they're very open." "A child doesn't distort the picture of his illness as much as an adult will do—there is less emotional overlay."

Dealing with children and psychiatric patients can be similar. Examinations for both are time consuming and often inconclusive. Information is difficult to get from children who may be fearful of the white-coated figure or who simply are not old enough to describe symptoms clearly; and emotionally ill patients often "ramble all around the subject" instead of answering questions directly. Although their rambling may itself be useful for diagnosis, it may unnerve you. Students frequently feel uncomfortable and unsure with emotionally disturbed patients and feel "even less confident" with them than with other patients. The combination of the patient's inability to communicate and the frustration of "having nothing I can put my hands on" can leave one feeling "helpless and ticked off in a lot of ways." Yet others prefer the subtle challenges presented by emotional illness.

Your early preferences for treating patients with acute or chronic illness may reflect your personality. Acutely ill patients offer more positive reinforcement than the chronically ill. "You can see the results of your treatment." "Acute illness is more exciting, more rewarding." "Somebody acutely ill you can treat. You can usually offer him something." But "the acutely ill patient has to be watched more closely and it's more time consuming and nerve racking." And, "at this stage of the game, I prefer chronic patients because I need to think about some of this stuff. With someone acutely ill, you need to know what you're doing and have some confidence."

Your choices for a particular gender and socioeconomic group reflect your own attitudes and probably won't change dramatically. For example, a male student may find it "easier to walk in and achieve rapport with a male patient." Some women insist that their male colleagues' sexist preferences are influenced by those who train them. And, as these male comments indicate, sexism does impact some student patient preferences: "Women seem to be a little more whiny and complaining. They have too many questions." "I don't care if I treat males or females as long as the females aren't on Gyn. Female patients have a certain neurotic personality once they get on that service—just screws up their whole attitude." "Men are more stable and have fewer psychological problems."

A definite stumbling block exists for male students with female patients. "You can't just walk in and examine them. You have to find a nurse to chaperon, and you feel like you're bothering the nurses when you ask them." Still, some men prefer to treat women because "female patients are more cooperative." "Women are nice and friendly—overall the nicest patients." But, as most students eventually discover, "There are no real differences between male and female patients. Some patients are difficult to deal with, regardless of gender. In general, I've found that I get back from the patient what I've put in—if I'm friendly and outgoing they tend to respond more cheerfully and appreciatively."

Some students who come to medical school with the plan to practice in an inner-city or rural community prefer treating economically disadvantaged patients. "Sure, it's nicer to examine a nice-looking, clean-smelling person, but I still want to work with needy people." These patients offer some advantages, at least for this student physician: "Their diseases are usually more advanced and interesting." "They're easier to work with than private patients because they tend to look on us as doctors. Private patients know we're students and it bothers them having us around; they know we're there for our own learning."

Clinical Activities

The third year introduces new and unexpected stressors. "Third year is very physically demanding, with much longer hours. It's like a job where you have to be there no matter what, even if you have the flu and feel lousy." For the first time, what you do as a medical student directly affects another human being. The fear of bad grades, the threat of failure, competition, financial dependency, and sexual deprivation may be constant throughout your medical school career, but probably not until your third year will you be exposed to chronic or terminal illness, a patient's death, a family's bereavement, or consequences of a medical error. "There's so much to learn. You just can't learn it all and I'm afraid I may miss some things and hurt someone."

Third-year students typically distance themselves from the emotions that accompany dying and death: "Suddenly, it occurred to me that I was instinctively shutting off my emotions to deal with the man's death. Was it supposed to be like that?" "It seems like this year I've become emotionally isolated from patients, which worries me at times." "I guess I have a somewhat-fatalistic attitude now." Third-year students, coming face to face with their limitations, are more accepting than first- and second-year students that "Sometimes nothing can be done," although this is still a bitter admission. "It's hard to view yourself as a doctor who has a responsibility to help people and yet to know you're more-or-less useless in many cases."

After pushing so hard during the first two years, some burned-out students experience a psychological letdown, and a few, depression. "After pushing so hard for so long, you have a natural urge to let down a little. I'm just tired." "I got very depressed, but not because I wasn't motivated. I felt that there were too many demands on us, which prevented me from studying and learning as I would like." Some seek supportive counseling: "I can't talk to my friends about it, so I've got to find a professional listener. I guess the best thing to do is to talk to a psychiatrist." By the end of the third year, however, you feel generally rewarded with increased status and confidence, a sense of doing what you imagined medical school to be—helping patients.

Diagnosis

After a few weeks on a clinical rotation, most students recognize at least the casebook examples of certain conditions. "I'm catching on quicker than I thought I would. I can get in the ballpark." "I usually understand what's going on with my patients, even when I'm not the first to pick it up." "I get pleasure out of making a diagnosis and go brag to my wife about it." You're still grateful not to have to act without guidance and support. "I can make a diagnosis sufficient not to let a person die from it, but I'm not quite ready to treat anyone." "I would never treat a patient on the basis of my own diagnosis."

As a third-year student, you suspect you'll never feel 100% confident of your ability. "I still have a hard time remembering the big kinds of drugs, let alone the little ones." "I don't know what I'm doing all the time, and it's so easy to make a mistake." Possibly, you'll be aware for the first time of diagnostic dilemmas that baffle even the more experienced clinicians. The humility that comes with awareness of personal limitations is one of the most valuable lessons learned in medical school: "I have a good deal of information, but I don't know how to apply it. The more you learn and the more you see, the more you realize you don't know very much." "When I get my MD and somebody tells me I'm a doctor, I'll start to feel confident. And that will be because somebody tells me so, not because I believe I know it all."

Physical Examinations

Students of both sexes are nervous about their first physical examinations. One student shares her experience:

> Finally the day of my first physical exam had arrived. . . . I remember reciting the procedures . . . over and over. . . . I arrived at the hospital with my group. . . . The six of us looked at one another one last loving time. The look was one of encouragement, support, and basically outright terror.

She was assigned to Mr. A., an obese person:

> I kept asking questions and listening to his answers . . . until I came to the topic of sex. I couldn't do it. . . . I could not bring myself to address this forbidden topic. . . . The physical examination part was truly a nightmare. . . . This man had body odor! . . . I tried to calm my fear that I was going to launch my lunch in Mr. A.'s lap.[9]

Male students usually feel incompetent when doing pelvic exams on female patients. "The first few times I didn't know what I was looking for. I just went through the motions and hoped I wasn't hurting her or showing how ill at ease I was." "At first, I didn't know the difference between normal and abnormal." Such examinations can be embarrassing for both parties. "The patient knows I'm a student and I'm embarrassed." And third-year students may face an additional problem by being the third or fourth person to examine the same patient. She may come "to feel like she's being molested or something," one worried.

Some men experience major anxiety about the sexual implications of examining female patients. "I have trouble dissociating the physician-patient relationship from the male-female relationship," one said. "I have a fear of getting dragged into court for something I never did. I've heard so much about it. I worry about what might happen after an examination."

One male student had this startling reaction:

> Looking up from the hospital bed was . . . this drop-dead gorgeous woman. Cupid shot me through the heart with his arrow. . . . I began to feel light-headed, as if I could actually sense any semblance of knowledge escaping through my ears. Wasn't it totally inappropriate, hell, downright illegal, for me to be feeling this way?[10]

Women medical students face different problems. Male physicians sometimes embarrass them by explaining or apologizing to male patients for the presence of a woman: "The young lady here is going to be a doctor."

Most women students describe their diagnostic experiences with males in terms of examinations of older patients.

> I haven't had to examine a man my own age yet, but you have to act straight—I'm here as a doctor, not a potential date. I think if you come on totally professional, they won't misinterpret. If they feel embarrassed and don't want you to examine them, I guess you get another doctor.

"It's interesting that some male patients do not want female doctors to examine them, although female nurses must handle them daily—putting in catheters, rectal temps, etc."

Like their male colleagues, women report that they are not specifically instructed how to conduct a physical exam on members of the opposite sex or how to deal with any problems. They are left to work it out on their own: "Nobody's ever said anything about how you handle it if a male patient doesn't want to take his pants off in front of you. It's something I'm going to have to figure out for myself." "I work at a VD clinic. You are never told how to deal with male patients when examining them; you just *do* it."

When I worked at the VA hospital, I got very accustomed to examining males, and there was sort of a standard comment when I'd come in. They'd say, "Well, I knew a student was going to examine me, but I didn't know it was going to be a pretty young lady." But I never had anybody actively resist or actively pursue me for a date.

Some students fear that learning to compartmentalize or suppress their sexual feelings might adversely affect their personal relationships, but others see no such problem. Some students use their spouses or significant others to practice their physical exams and have no loss of amorous feelings as a result. In fact, for third-year students, as for first- and second-year students, the greatest impediment to romance is not familiarity but exhaustion!

Insights: Active Listening
Bernard Virshup, MD

One of the most exciting and critical events in your life as a medical student is when you introduce yourself to your first patient to take a history. You are apt to have a lot of feelings about this. "How well will I handle this interview?" "What will the patient think of me?" "What will my instructor think?" This is called "white-coat anxiety," for many students feel like frauds wearing the coat; what if the patient, thinking you are a real doctor, asks you something you don't know? What if you run out of questions and can't think of anything else to ask?

There is a tool that, properly used, can relieve much of this concern and turn every interview into something wonderful and enjoyable—for you and your patient. It is called active listening.

No doubt, you have seen a child, filled with some great emotion, struggle to tell his or her mother about what happened, while the mother, adopting the same expression as the child, waits with love and patience until the little one finds just the right words. It is through experiences like this that bonding occurs. This child, knowing he or she is loved, will grow up feeling secure. The need to feel important—heard, understood, and affirmed—does not go away when we grow up, especially when we become patients. Every patient experiences anxiety and a loss of control. When we become ill, we need to be mothered, to be listened to, to be reassured. A clinician's active listening fulfills these needs.

There are many components of active listening, but I suggest you focus on mirroring and reflecting.

Mirroring

When talking with others, many of us allow ourselves unconsciously and naturally to mirror the other's body language—the posture, expression, and gestures by which all of us express ourselves and that tell so much about us. By mirroring, we understand better who another person is, what he or she is about, what he or she is feeling. Even more important, the other feels understood and affirmed by the person doing the mirroring, often without understanding why. The person doing the mirroring sends out a nonverbal message to the other of understanding and acceptance, and without really being aware of what is happening the other person begins to trust and to share thoughts and feelings. For me, empathy is the feeling you get within you when you allow yourself to mirror another person. When you adopt the other's posture and expression, you find yourself experiencing what the other person experiences. You begin to know, to accept, and to admire the other person.

Reflection

Active listening also involves reflection, repeating one or more of the other's words, thoughts, or feelings, perhaps rephrasing them to focus them. When added to mirroring, reflection is a powerful stimulus for promoting further self-disclosure and meaningful closeness. At first, reflection might seem awkward to you. Most people who are good at it sincerely want to hear more of what the other has to say and don't want to intrude their own ideas into the other's thoughts. Repeating a word or a phrase assures the other person that you are interested in what he or she is saying and encourages the person to say more. It stimulates the other to think more and delve deeper into a subject he or she has already indicated willingness to share with you.

Some people find it difficult to listen in such an empathic way. Carl Rogers once wrote that it is very difficult for people to permit themselves to understand others. "Is it necessary to permit ourselves to understand another?" he asked.[11] I think it is. Our first reaction to most of the statements we hear from other people is an immediate evaluation or judgment: That's right, that's stupid, that's unreasonable. Very rarely do we permit ourselves to understand precisely what the meaning of the statement is to the person making it. When you are open to the thoughts and feelings of others, you must have tools for dealing with them when they are disturbing. What is one to do with the other person's feelings?

Here is another tool: Reach out and touch the other's hand while making affirming and understanding noises.

What you should not do is immediately try to "fix" the other. We often want to help others by telling them they shouldn't feel this way, by giving advice, or by showing a better way. *Don't!* It is usually counterproductive. Most people just want you to be there and to understand.

Knowing this makes it much easier to listen to people when they are telling you about their problems and feelings. You really don't have to do anything. For the physician, active listening is an important skill—sometimes even more important than the ability to ask the "right questions." To make an intelligent differential diagnosis, the physician needs a lot of information, which he or she normally obtains by asking questions. But questions sometimes get in the way of active listening, of patient self-disclosure, of intimacy. It is hard to do both. Very often, questions will be unnecessary; the patient will supply the important information without being asked, if the physician only waits a little longer. Very often, the physician can use reflection of a significant word or phrase to channel the flow of words, and this helps the patient explore the symptom or situation appropriately, without questions being necessary at all. The skilled physician knows when to actively and patiently listen to the patient and when finally to step in with crucial questions that may cut off the flow of further information.

One of the most difficult things for the neophyte student to deal with is silence. It is common for the patient to look at the student and wait for the next question. Then, you feel the pressure to respond by thinking of another question to ask. It is important that you learn to resist this urge. This itself is an important lesson: Discomfort need not be immediately relieved by action.

With active listening, patients will generally give you the information you need, very quickly. They may even flood you with information. Then, your challenge will be to direct this flow, by repeating crucial words in the direction you want to go. When students learn to conduct an interview without more than three or four questions, they become much less anxious, more comfortable with patients, and more confident of their ability to conduct an interview and to achieve closeness with their patient.

The trusting doctor-patient relationship is established in the first few minutes—otherwise not at all or with great difficulty. A good doctor-patient relationship is based not on physician competence but on the perception that the doctor listens, understands, and cares. This is achieved by active listening:

mirroring, accurate reflection, and responding appropriately to the patient's feelings.

Notes

1. Blain, Arthur. 1997, March. "Friday Night in a South Bronx ER." *The New Physician,* p. 33.

2. Fink, Randy A. 1996, July-August. "The Great Pretender." *The New Physician,* p. 41.

3. Fugh-Berman, Adriane. n.d. "Relative Realities." *The New Scope* (Georgetown University School of Medicine Student News).

4. Lawlor, Danny. 1987, March. "Third Year: An Introduction to the Hierarchy." *The New Scope* (Georgetown University School of Medicine Student News).

5. Whitaker, Eric E. 1992, January-February. "Stress: An Avoidable Hazard." *The New Physician,* p. 47.

6. Sargeant, Risa R. 1995, Summer. "A Patient in the Teaching Hospital: Balancing Privacy and Education." *The Pharos,* pp. 29-34, p. 33.

7. *Ibid.,* p. 31.

8. *Ibid.,* p. 33.

9. Gujrathi, Sheila. 1996, Winter. "Intimate Strangers." *The Pharos,* pp. 34-35.

10. Reifler, Douglas R. 1996, Winter. "Early Patient Encounters: Second-Year Student Narratives of Initiation Into Clinical Medicine." *The Pharos,* pp. 29-33, p. 31.

11. Rogers, Carl. 1961. *On Becoming A Person.* Boston: Houghton Mifflin.

Challenging Issues
What If I Make a Mistake?

We physicians are even less prepared to deal with our own mistakes than the average lay person is. The climate of medical school and residency training, for instance, makes it nearly impossible to confront the emotional consequences of mistakes.[1]

—Family physician

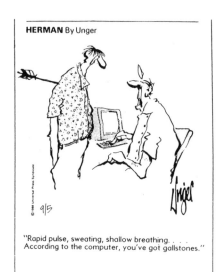

HERMAN By Unger

"Rapid pulse, sweating, shallow breathing. . . . According to the computer, you've got gallstones."

You will make mistakes. Don't burden yourself with unrealistic expectations of perfection. I know of one surgery resident who committed suicide after one of his mentors reprimanded him in the surgery suite for dropping an instrument. Sleep deprived and rigidly controlled, he regarded himself a failure, a misfit in medicine.

Unfortunately, errors in medicine are rarely acknowledged or openly discussed except in public morbidity and mortality conferences or in post-mortem clinical pathology conferences. Many times, the physician who made the mistake feels spotlighted for ridicule when the technical details are discussed. Everyone leaves with the idea that if one had been smart and conscientious enough, the patient would still be alive. Actually, errors occur everyday. Despite your best intentions and efforts, you will make your share.

You will confront other challenging issues. How will you deal with contagion and with annoying or critically ill patients without making matters worse? What will you say to the loved ones of those who die? Be open to learning how to handle these and other challenging situations throughout your career. Learn from your own mistakes and those of others. Be honest with yourself and, most important, remember that you don't need to be perfect.

Medical Errors

Newspaper and television reports of hospital errors have made the public more aware of medical mistakes, such as using the wrong X ray or amputating the wrong foot. Dr. Lucien Leape of the Harvard School of Public Health estimates that each year about 1.3 million people experience an injury related to medical treatment. About 180,000 people die as a result of injuries and about half are probably related to error.[2]

When Dr. David Bates and his colleagues looked at the frequency of drug errors in two prominent Boston hospitals, they found 6.5 drug complications for every 100 admissions. The major problems were (a) physicians ordering the wrong dosage, (b) incorrect copies of the drug order, (c) pharmacies dispensing the wrong drug, and (d) nurses administering drugs to the wrong patient. These errors, they say, were ordinary, the kind made every day. "How many times have you written down a telephone number and gotten one of the digits wrong?" Leape inquires. "But when that happens with a medication order, or dispensing a prescription, it can have serious effects."[3]

In a forum that discussed this issue, Dr. Nancy Dickey criticized Bates's remarks, noting that the average patient probably takes between 5 and 15 different drugs. "The fact that they found only 247 errors is unbelievable, considering the number of interactions that occur with each of those patients every day."[4]

In his classic book, *Healing the Wounds,* Dr. David Hilfiker openly discusses the mistakes he made as a private practitioner. "Everyone, of course, makes mistakes," he acknowledges.

> But the potential consequences of our medical mistakes are so overwhelming that it is almost impossible for practicing physicians to deal with their errors in a psychologically healthy fashion. Most people—doctors and patients alike—harbor deep within themselves the expectation that the physician will be perfect. No one seems prepared to accept the simple fact of life that physicians, like anyone else, will make mistakes.[5]

The teaching hospital is "an environment in which precision seems to predominate," Hilfiker points out:

> When the physician does make an important mistake it is first whispered about in the halls, as if it were a sin. Much later, a case conference is called in which experts who have had weeks to think about the situation discuss the way it should have been handled. The environment in which physicians are trained does not encourage them to talk about their mistakes or about the emotional responses to them.[6]

"The retrospective view is always 20/20 vision."

Sadly, in the medical environment, mistakes are too often seen not only as harmful to patients but as personal failure, a devastating assault on one's fragile ego. For example, when a college professor died after prostate surgery due to botched procedures, the surgeon told the wife and children, "For you this is unpleasant, awful; but believe me, for me it's shattering."[7]

Contagion

Students on medical services where they contact infectious diseases understandably worry about contagion. "Getting sick is a real threat. You're worn down and therefore more susceptible; you're exposed frequently and more aware of the potential dire consequences of certain diseases."

Married students, especially those with small children at home, are particularly sensitive to the dangers of contracting or transmitting a disease. "I think of my little girl coming up on my lap when I have a lab coat on. I worry about there being something on it to infect her." "I had a patient with typhoid and I didn't spend as much time there as I should have. I was afraid of it."

A few decades ago, medical students felt impervious to disease and adopted a somewhat cavalier attitude. No longer. AIDS has rendered serious risk an all-too-real possibility. "The decision to go into medicine takes on a soul-searching dimension, because you are literally dealing with a deadly and infectious disease on an almost daily basis."

Historically, the general populace shuns those stricken with serious, incurable infectious diseases. At the turn of the 20th century, the United States experienced a general hysteria about syphilis and gonorrhea.[8] Physicians suggested that people could contract what they labeled "casually transmitted venereal diseases" through everyday activities, without sexual contact. And they cataloged the various ways that syphilis, for example, might be communicated, such as touching a pen, pencil, or toothbrush. When physicians became infected, it was generally assumed it was a result of performing surgical procedures on patients with venereal disease. These beliefs, of course, no longer prevail.

People formerly shunned cancer patients as if it was transmitted through casual contact. Most avoidance behavior now focuses on Acquired Immunodeficiency Syndrome (AIDS), a disease that strongly impacts the way Americans live, interact, and regard other people.

An emergency room physician relates that a demented AIDS patient inadvertently disconnected his IV line. Blood dribbled from the tube, covering the walls and floor of his room; the doctor gingerly reconnected the tubing and called housekeeping to come clean up the mess. But no one would respond. "After much arguing, a man arrived with a mop, wearing a suit that looked as if it were made for nuclear decontamination. In contrast to our paranoia about treating AIDS patients," this physician notes, "we blithely treated other people without taking any precautions at all. If they didn't belong to a risk group, we assumed they couldn't have the virus and we frequently drew their blood barehanded."[9]

One study of health profession students found that most of the students (71.2%) believed they were jeopardizing their own health by working with AIDS patients.[10] Elisabeth Rosenthal acknowledges that AIDS impacted residency selections of many of her classmates:

> I knew I wanted to return home to New York City, but AIDS was already changing the face of medical training in the country's urban centers, and many classmates would not even consider excellent programs in a place like New York and San Francisco. We like to say that our concern was purely academic: good medical training requires seeing a wide spectrum of diseases. How much could we learn if (as was sometimes the case during my internship) 20% of our patients had the same disease? Our real concern was often more personal. Many of us balked at the prospect of watching patients, often no older than ourselves, die miserably of what then seemed like a thoroughly hopeless disease. . . . [Also] the odds of an occasional, accidental needle stick are very high; I don't know of anyone I trained with who hasn't been pierced by using a needle.[11]

In a 1992 study reported by Michele Turk, 25%-80% of medical trainees injure themselves in the first year of clinical training.[12] Almost half of the recent graduates at the University of Washington School of Medicine reported having a needle stick injury or being splashed with infectious fluids during their third-and fourth-year clinical rotations.

It ia reported that health care workers are accidentally stuck about 800,000 times every year, 15% of them while disposing of needles and syringes. Of these health care workers, 12,000 annually become infected with hepatitis B and 200 to 300 die.[13] Students who have been infected with the HIV virus, says an observer interviewed by Turk, face a number of dilemmas:

> Do I keep silent or do I jeopardize my career? Do I go into surgery because I have always wanted to and risk unemployment, or do I enter something I like less? Do I stay near my family in South Carolina or go to New York and California where the climate is better for HIV-positive health care workers?[14]

There is much underreporting: "There is a huge disincentive for healthcare workers to report their injuries or seropositivity," said a physician who personally talked to more than 32 health care workers who became HIV positive on the job. "They're afraid of losing their job, their insurance, their family and their life."[15]

Shatz, executive director of the American Association of Physicians for Human Rights (AAPHR), advises students against disclosing that they are HIV positive unless they feel a moral obligation or are legally required to do so. Revealing one's status, he asserts, may bring their education to an abrupt end. He knows of several students and residents who were kicked out because they are HIV positive. On the other hand, if they do not disclose their problem, they may have difficulty getting treatment. Medical insurance also poses a problem for HIV-positive students since this condition hinders their ability to get new coverage.[16]

Susan Boyd, a psychiatry intern, describes her fear, anxious voices that argued within her when she accidentally stuck an IV needle in her index finger. "Putting the stylet back on the table (*like we are supposed to!*), I had rammed it into my finger."[17] Trying to appear calm and casual in front of her patient, she inwardly panicked, "I'll get AIDS!" "There was a chorus of hysterical voices elbowing their way into my consciousness":

> If I get AIDS, I'll deal with it. (*No I won't*). I'm not going to get AIDS, because this is a low-risk patient (*Yes, I will*). Better call the needlestick hotline first. I'm negative. Retest in six weeks. Use condoms. Don't do-

nate blood. Try not to worry. The needlestick nurse says people lie awake nights checking their lymph nodes. I've got to stay calm. The odds are with me. One in 250. Six-week recheck. Anonymously, at the health department. At student health, it's "confidential." Confidential can mean a lot of things. "Known only to one," or "known to a small army." The nurse's hand shakes as she spears me with a 16-gauge harpoon they use to draw blood. Negative at six weeks. The health department counselor breaks the rules and tells me over the phone. Professional courtesy. I thank God and make a prayer involving a promise never to do stupid or dangerous things and to always know what my left hand is doing. I volunteer to be reharpooned at three months.[18]

Fortunately, most internships and residencies have a confidential needle-stick service.

I stabbed myself with a lumbar puncture needle used on an AIDS patient with HIV dementia at about midnight on one of my busiest call nights as an intern. I didn't have time to panic, because I also had other patients to attend. I did go to the ED [Emergency Department], and everyone from the nurses on through the ranks of physicians came forward with a personal needle-stick story that had a happy ending. I was efficiently tested for and immunized against hepatitis that night, and the next day, our specialist nurse practitioner contacted me to counsel me on what was next. It wasn't until I got home the next day that I started to panic about how my career might have a premature ending, then how I should break off my engagement, and how worried and upset my parents would be. Thank goodness, my fiance had already talked to his infectious disease consultant, who reassured us that the probability of converting to HIV+ was very low.

I eventually tested negative for the third time (Day 1, Month 3, Month 6, Year 1) and could relax, but in the meantime I found a lot of support from my colleagues and coworkers. Now, I'm one of the staff who comes forward when someone else in training gets stuck with a needle.

Technology can eliminate about 85% of all needle-stick injuries. But these safety products are not in regular use, mostly because of their expense. Some needles, for instance, cost up to 20 times as much as traditional devices.[19] Some hospitals have a 24-hour hotline that workers can call to report an injury or receive counseling for the stress of potential AIDS virus infection from a needle-stick injury.

What is the risk of acquiring AIDS in the health care setting? "In all," Koelbl says, "the evidence still prevails that casual contact, including contact by dental professionals and other health-care workers, with AIDS-infected individuals does not incur a significant risk for HIV transmission."[20]

Sometimes, the situation is reversed and a clinician infects a patient. Recent studies show that a patient's chance of contracting the AIDS virus from a doctor or dentist is remote: "Thousands of patients were treated by a surgeon, a family practitioner who handled obstetrics and gynecology cases, and a dentist, all of whom were infected, without contracting the virus."[21] The Centers for Disease Control estimate that the probability of a known HIV-positive surgeon infecting his or her patients is 1 in 41,667 to 1 in 416,667. The risk for dentists is one in 263,158 to one in 2,631,579.[22]

But it does happen. The *Los Angeles Times* reported that an unnamed surgery resident at the UCLA Medical Center transmitted hepatitis B infection to 13% of the 144 patients he operated on during one year. Small cuts on his hands that he incurred while operating and leaks in his gloves passed on his own virus-laden blood. It is the only documented U.S. outbreak of hepatitis B linked to a thoracic surgeon (but other outbreaks have been documented in the United Kingdom).[23]

Aggravating Patients

Some patients are pleasant, cooperative, and grateful. Others are demanding, rude, or overly talkative. Some interruptions are justifiable, but it's annoying when patients invade your personal time for minor or trivial reasons. In such cases, you may tell them, as some seasoned veterans do, that you will return their call when you have their records available. "We have patients who call and beep every time they feel anything," a cardiologist complained:

> In a lot of situations, I have to tell them they are unduly anxious compared to others with the same problem, and that it will take a toll mentally and physically if they don't learn to deal with it. In some cases I suggest they talk to a psychiatrist about resolving their anxiety.[24]

Some patients generate other mundane but pesky problems. They may not respect the physician's schedule by coming late or rescheduling appointments three or four times. Nonpaying patients can be very grateful until they receive the bill; then they claim the doctor hasn't done anything to help them. "It's amazing how the medical bill changes their entire outlook," one physician said.[25] Many doctors turn to collection agencies when they are stuck with a delinquent account. Others interpret delinquency of payment as a measure of their personal failure as healers. Payment complicates the doctor-patient relationship by raising issues of self-worth, politics, patient satisfaction, codependency, and survival.

Unhygienic patients with severe body odor are unpleasant to treat. "Sometimes it seems as though it has been a month since their last bath," one clinician complained. "I have to hold my breath and spray the room after they leave."[26]

Patients who have a psychological need to be ill may become abusive and antagonistic. They have usually been to several other doctors—"doctor shopping"—and nobody has told them what they want to hear. Calling these patients "symptom magnifiers," Samuel Greengard says they feign or exaggerate their problems, sometimes to collect insurance or disability payments and drag things out for their own financial advantage.[27] These patients appear in all clinical settings—at county general clinics and at private practitioners' offices.

Drug and alcohol abusers are difficult to treat because they tend to be extremely manipulative. Frequent telephone calls from them can strain credulity:

> I have people tell me, "The cat knocked the pill bottle into the toilet." When you mention coming into the office, they have instant diarrhea and can't possibly leave the bathroom. They always have an excuse or justification no matter what you suggest to help besides giving them the desired drug script.

One physician recounts that a drug-abusing woman called his office 12 times in one day:

> The office staff told her I would call her back later, but she kept calling with increasingly terrible symptoms. She said that a horrible sore had popped up on her breast and it needed urgent attention. As it turned out this gigantic sore turned into a little pimple that had popped and was just fine.[28]

Noncompliant patients often frustrate the physician. One doctor developed and proposed a comprehensive strategy to deal with a patient's breast cancer. She had a realistic chance of surviving but decided that she would go home and surrender to God's will. Other patients exacerbate their condition by not following the doctor's recommendations. "Unfortunately there is only so much you can do," one physician said. "And the rest is up to them. Trying to change behaviors is the most difficult thing to do."[29] Of course, there may be another side of this story: Maybe the expectations are unrealistic or instructions weren't clear.

What should you tolerate? Most physicians set boundaries and occasionally dismiss a patient for noncompliance nonpayment. "When the patient is hostile and doesn't want to follow instructions, I tell them it would be better to go somewhere else," one said.[30] "You may be required by law to provide the patient with the names of other physicians they can go to and then give them 30 days before ending your relationship."

You will develop your own coping style with difficult patients. Keep in mind that it's important to assess patients' psychological as well as physical needs. In so doing, you will take a big step toward treating them effectively. But establish boundaries and realize that some patients may be beyond your effectiveness and patience.

When annoying patients drain your precious time and energy, how can you express your frustration without getting into trouble with a training system that encourages denial and repression? Here's when medical slang may be useful, because it provides an acceptable way to discharge resentments and other strong emotions. Slang terms deflect feelings of anger, disgust, and frustration that are incompatible with those formally defined as appropriate, (e.g., compassion). It provides a safety valve for letting off steam, a way to criticize patients who create seemingly unnecessary stress for you. A resident physician explained, "Humorous, often sarcastic slang terms provide an outlet for our stress, a socially acceptable outlet, whereas being uptight and rude to our patients is not."[31]

A patient who is frustrating because his or her condition cannot be diagnosed is called a "crock." Although the term is not said in their presence, "nutty" patients may be called "squirrel bait." "Gomer" refers to patients who lack wit or social status, usually senile, chronically ill, or noncompliant ones. A "troll" is a patient who is a pain in the neck, such as an old, debilitated, or sometimes incontinent man. A patient with a combination of medical problems incompatible with survival may be called a "train wreck"—one problem worsens as a result of treatment for another—and one unconscious and likely to stay that way is "gorked" (*G*od *O*nly *R*eally *K*nows) or "circling the drain." Although these terms may now sound heartless and insensitive, you will probably use them if they provide relief in pressure situations. Slang is also a means to communicate privately about sensitive topics in the presence of patients and their families.

Critically Ill Patients

When you work in the emergency room, the intensive care unit (ICU), or other similar settings with critically ill or injured patients, you will be challenged to maintain composure in the face of emotional crisis.[32] On the one hand, you must not overly identify with your patients but remain somewhat emotionally detached, and on the other, you must stay compassionate and caring. How will you react to emotionally charged situations?

The ICU, for example, can be a particularly dramatic and intense setting. The work necessitates constant watchfulness, and frequent crises require prompt and aggressive action. There is no room for hesitation due to insecurities about one's skill or knowledge. Patients are fearful; concerned family members haunt the corridors; and health providers are often fatigued, impatient, and hypercritical. Labeled "Death Valley" by some, the ICU contains a constantly pulsing and humming assortment of technical equipment crowded into a relatively small space with critically ill or postoperative patients. These patients can be querulous and demanding if they are not intubated, and it may be necessary to employ one pain-inflicting measure after another—establishing multiple IV accesses, turning, deep breathing, changing dressings, and so on. How will you maintain a proper balance between sympathy and objectivity? Here are some ways to cope.

Escape Into Work

Constant work activity often supplants other coping mechanisms. When you are very busy, you can immerse yourself in the technical tasks at hand rather than absorb the emotions around you. For example, a seriously injured patient loudly moaning will not disturb the staff's tranquility if they keep very busy. "Most of the staff were so busy they did not have time to think about or hear the moaning," observed a medical student. "I noticed that the only time I was bothered by it was when I sat down for awhile."

Rationalization

When death appears imminent, you may find rationalization useful. Death can be explained, for example, as a welcome relief from the suffering caused by the patient's illness. Talking in advance of the death allows clinicians to prepare themselves for the emotional repercussions. When a child is about to die, for example, the staff may go about its business in a normal matter. "Most had already accepted the fact that the child just didn't have a chance and had already prepared themselves for the event."

Humor

Humor, one of the most common techniques used to "manage" emotional stress, occurs in joking, kidding, and good-natured ribbing among clinical staff. "Small things are called to attention in order to make fun of them," observed a student. All members of the ICU staff, especially the more experienced, take part in the effort to keep the atmosphere as light as possible. When a staff member becomes too serious, others try to involve him in the lighthearted banter. Sometimes, patients are also drawn into the joking. After listening to the groaning of the semiconscious patients for a long time, a clinician said to a neighboring patient, "If you start hollering, we can start a chorus." They both laughed and a joke developed between doctors and patients.

Lightheartedness in the midst of such painful human drama might seem inappropriate to some observers, but joking around does not appear to interfere with doing a good job. If anything, it contributes to the quality of work performance since it reduces the emotional strain created by the constant stream and demands of critically ill patients. When a nursing supervisor complained that there was too much "clowning" on the unit, another responded, "You couldn't work in this place without laughing or you'd go crazy."

Language Alteration

Clinical personnel prefer the terms "arrest" or "cardiac arrest" to "heart attack" because the latter is a layperson's term—misleading, uninformative, imprecise, or simply unscientific. But it is also less stressful to use "trade" terms. The technical terms isolate the suffering by classifying it as a medical event—an event that occurs in professional life rather than in personal life—and thus permit easier and freer discussion.

Indirect speech also softens reference to stressful events. "The situation" or "the incident" refers to death. During stressful times, speech tends to become vague, oblique, and allusive. This vagueness also avoids anxiety that might be created by overly bold or frequent references to death.

Similarly, euphemisms can obscure the event. ICU personnel speak about those who are "not going to make it" or are "on a hopeless decline." "Critically ill," although not a euphemism, functions as one to avoid referring to a patient as "dying."

Latin-derived terms also reduce stress and make discussion of difficult subjects easier. "To perish" or to "expire" are identical in meaning to "die," but neither term has the immediacy or emotional force of the Anglo-Saxon.[33] As George Orwell stated, "Inflated style is in of itself a kind of euphemism. A mass of Latin words falls upon the facts like soft snow, blurring the outlines and covering up all the details."[34]

As already discussed, slang, like euphemisms and technical terms, veils the harsh realities of medical life. When stressful conditions threaten to physically and emotionally overburden physicians, medical slang helps them deal with their feelings. "Even the nicest doctor uses slang terms because they allow him to feel superior, even if he's losing the battle over the patient's disease; they make him feel better."[35]

Slang terms communicate when a patient's condition is grave. "If a patient is really at the end of the road," one physician explained, "'We'll just say, 'He showed the dotted Q sign this morning,' and everyone knows what you mean." The facial features of patients in the last few days of life frequently approximate the letter Q—mouth open, tongue hanging to the side.[36]

Patients afflicted with terminal illnesses may have their diagnosis disguised with slang terms such as "the Big A" (AIDS), "the Big C" (cancer), or other slang terms such as "Crunchcase" (head injury), "failure to fly" (injuries caused by a fall), "failure to float" (a near drowning). Motorcycle riders frequently in and out of hospitals are called "organ donors."

Again, it's important to realize that slang terms do not necessarily express insensitivity or lack of concern for patients, but they usually relieve tension and provide coded communication. "I had heard some slang terms before I started school and I never thought I would use them. They do sound cold. But when you're in the situation day after day, you learn to get to the point and a word or phrase can sum up a patient." Together with concentration on work, rationalization, humor and other language alteration, medical slang enables caregivers to maintain emotional balance in emotionally trying and intense situations.

Death

Once exposed to dying patients, you will probably reevaluate your attitudes about life and death and eventually recognize that sometimes you can not keep a patient from dying. "A few weeks ago, I realized for the first time that there was absolutely no way that I or anybody else could help this patient, and I was really depressed most of the time."

Some cases are particularly poignant. "I had a little girl with leukemia," one said, "and I got to where I didn't even want to go into the room to see her."

> When it's a kid, maybe eight years old, it really gets you. With an older person—like a chronic-lunger who just moped around and never took his medicine—it's different. He wouldn't do anything for himself and became a real pain in the neck. When he died, we felt like he deserved it.

You may develop a close relationship with a dying patient: "I had one patient, a 26-year-old from the upper middle class who was intelligent and pretty; we had similar backgrounds and expectations. I had stronger feelings for her and her husband than for any other patient I'd taken care of."

You might question the ethics of keeping dying patients alive. "It's a crummy feeling when patients you know are going to die. You're prolonging a life and wonder if you should." "They're keeping him alive with respirators, and I'm leaning toward the side of, 'Just let the poor guy die.'"

As a third-year student you'll develop a new familiarity with death. Is it an enemy to be fought at all costs? Perhaps without being conscious of your changing attitudes, you'll begin to react differently to death. This will be just one of the ways you will grow into your new role. You also move one more step out of the realm of laypersons and settle a bit more firmly into a new world in which disability and death are daily events.

Medical trainees typically, but not inevitably, evolve through fairly predictable developmental stages in dealing with death.

Stage 1: Idealizing the Doctor's Role

Entering students, like the general public, regard the doctor as a bulwark against suffering and death. "That's my business," one said, "to make sure that death doesn't occur."

Idealistic students may be offended by the coolness of a case-hardened clinician. A first-year student who accompanied an upper-division student on rounds was appalled by the "unfeeling way" the attending physician talked to the group about a terminally ill patient. "I'd sure hate to have a family here and talk like that," he said. "I suppose the doctor has to be uncompassionate at times, but I wasn't ready for it. He wasn't disrespectful, but he just didn't show any emotion."

Similarly, a second-year student was shocked by the detached attitude of the staff when his first patient died. Unaware of her death, he entered her room and was told matter of factly, "She's in the morgue." "This really bothered me," he related. "I went to her autopsy and it made me think pretty deeply for a long while."

The scientific interest displayed by clinical staff in a patient's demise dismays some students. When a surgical team dispassionately discussed a baby who died during unsuccessful cardiac surgery, a student commented, "The surgeon was sorry, I guess, but it was kind of a scientific study to him; things like this evidently happen to him every week or two." Then, during the autopsy, the student was stunned when the pediatric cardiologist became excited to find the autopsy findings compared well with his own diagnosis of the case.

Although this detachment is disquieting, most students realize it does not necessarily indicate a lack of concern but at times is in the best interests of the patient. Later on, these same students find themselves reacting to death much like these mentors. But at the initial stage, they typically respond as laypersons.

Stage 2: Desensitizing Death Symbols

When you confront your cadaver during the first week of school, you will begin to learn emotional aloofness. Prospective doctors become desensitized to death's symbols—bones, blood, corpses, and stench—symbols that disturb most people. Some students became desensitized earlier during premed courses that required them to dissect or even kill living things. In any event, this phase of medical school can still be disturbing. A psychiatrist who interviewed students found that many of them had nightmares about their anatomy experiences.[37]

No matter how great the initial shock, however, it apparently wears off for most students. Before long, you may become so desensitized that you can eat lunch around the corpse. Medical students strive to look nonchalant and "cool" to make the anatomy experience tolerable.

You may utilize a number of coping mechanisms. Humor, previously mentioned, is a ready tension release. Although faculty discourage pranks and horseplay, amusing stories about the cadavers circulate among classmates who create clever names for the lifeless forms or arrange the body in such a way as to elicit a laugh. This all goes toward helping you forget the morose aspects of the task at hand.

The challenge to the prospective doctor is, of course, to keep personal sensitivities intact while dissecting a human body. Most derive inner relief by concentrating on the details of the work, by occupying themselves with the finite details of the dissection process and memorizing the scientific names of bones, muscles, nerves, and other body parts. Dissection then becomes a mechanical exercise rather than a humanistic experience. This absorption in work acts, in Harold Lief and Renee Fox's term, as "a psychic non-irritant."[38]

Usually during the second year, you will be introduced to pathology and experience your first autopsy. Here, you will respond much the same way you did with your cadaver. But autopsies will bring you much closer to the subjective aspects of death. Because the body was living only a few hours earlier, it is much more difficult to avoid identifying with the deceased. The body is less heavily draped than cadavers and appears much more lifelike. It is soft and has normal coloration and real, nonchemical smells. You may also know the patient's identity and medical history, read their chart, or listen to the doctor's report about the fatal illness.

So, to maintain equanimity and protect yourself from discomfort, you, like your mentors, will likely adopt a detached scientific attitude, suppressing your emotions by focusing on the technical aspects. Thinking about diseased tissues is less emotionally involving than remembering the patient as a person. Absorption in the pathological details of an autopsy will help you maintain the proper professional response—objectivity.

Constant exposure to scientific terminology in basic science courses will also desensitize you to the disease process, the precursor to death. "It is just hours and hours of looking at slides of people who have various illnesses at progressive stages," a physician recalled. "After a while, it just doesn't have the same emotional punch." In short, the basic science years will condition you psychologically to deal with the symbols of death in an unemotional way and to display the expected professional response—calm, objective, rational, and controlled emotions. This conditioning will prepare you for encounters with living patients.

Stage 3: Objectifying and Combating Death

When you leave the lecture room and laboratory for the hospital floors, you will witness some of life's most poignant dramas. Omnipresent are death's companions—pain, suffering, fear, and despair. Here, you will learn to distance yourself emotionally from the living as well as the dead. "It's really hard the first two or three times a patient dies," a fourth-year student explains, "so you learn to develop a protective shield to reduce the emotional impact":

> My first patient was a little boy suffering from incurable leukemia. He was all right when he left the hospital, but in about two weeks he came into the emergency room in shock and died three hours later. When I was in the room with him, the attending physician asked, "Who had this patient before?" When I told him I had, he sent me to look after the mother who was crying in the next room. While the doctor worked on the little five-year-old, I tried to talk to the mother. I really felt terribly inadequate; there wasn't a whole lot I could say to make her feel better. Then, we went into the room where they were treating the boy. He was screaming and crying and then stopped breathing. The mother collapsed and somebody caught her. That experience really got to me![39]

The main depersonalizing technique, modeled effectively by the clinical faculty, is to objectify death by denying its subjective features, that is, viewing the dying patient not as a person but as a medical entity and then concentrating only on the pathological part. "This is the old scientific fragmentalization method," one explained. "You just bust up the human organism into pieces and only deal with the pieces, then you don't have to see the whole picture." The patient then becomes "The liver in Room 212."

By adopting a scientific frame of mind, utilized in your previous work with cadavers, you may be able to mitigate uncomfortable inner feelings that occur when you are exposed to a dying patient. Then, as a fourth-year student explained, "Death can be as neutral as reading the obituary section of the newspaper."

This is not to say that doctors regard their clinical responsibilities lightly. On the contrary, there is every expectation that you will exhaust every possible technique to keep your patients alive. Before a person dies, there is usually a "mad scramble," as one student puts it, to do everything possible to save the patient. When breathing or the heart stops, an emergency announcement in code language comes over the public address system ("Code Blue, Room 227," for example). Available clinicians are expected to rush to the bedside of the dying patient. Special emergency squads race through the halls and the patient is hooked up to monitors and life-saving machinery that emit a variety of visual and auditory signals. "It's a frantic, noisy, confused state," one student said. "People in white clothing hurry about knocking themselves out to keep the patient alive." Only when every life-saving recourse is exhausted, do they let up. Extraordinary efforts to revive patients are routine in the hospital.

Morbidity and mortality conferences, called "M&M" or "death rounds," provide a forum for praising a job well done or criticizing a haphazard clinical performance. Whenever a patient dies, interns, residents, attending staff, and others gather together to discuss "the case." Whoever was responsible for the patient reviews the clinical history and the pathology report is given. Then, a discussion ensues on what could have been done differently to avoid the death. "This gave me the idea," one resident said, "that if we were just smarter and had not made this or that mistake the patient would still be alive." The assumption is that death is preventable and doesn't happen to patients of good physicians. At least, this is the idea that is "handed down" to medical trainees. No wonder physicians usually experience a sense of personal defeat when someone dies.

In short, at this stage of training, death is viewed as the enemy, the opponent waiting to snatch away the patient. "The whole idea of medical training," said one student, "is to teach doctors how to avoid death at almost any cost." So, the battle lines are drawn, with death in darkly mortal combat with white-attired physicians. At stake is the patient's life, as well as the clinician's reputation and self-esteem. "It's a shame somebody has to die," one student remarked. "I didn't become a doctor to see people die."

Stage 4: Questioning the Medical Model

Recognizing that teaching in some medical centers tends to dehumanize the patient and make technicians out of doctors, some thoughtful physicians question the glorification of the science of medicine. "I hate to admit it," one physician said, "but I had come to view the patient almost as an extension of all the apparatus." In this way, the social, emotional, and spiritual context of the dying person is overlooked and their death is treated as a technical event—when brain activity ceases, when respiratory and cardiac functions end, and when consciousness fades.

One physician reflected that he had become so imbued with the idea of combatting death that medical practice had become "a contest between me and the disease; the patient was merely an object over which we were fighting." When death is viewed as the enemy, one can justify extremes in prolonging life. "He's not about to let his omnipotence be challenged if he can help it," a physician remarked about a colleague. "But if you talk to the family, you will find that they are usually sorry that the patient had to suffer those extra days and that the hospital bill ran up so high."

Some physicians and the public question whether efforts to avoid death at any cost are appropriate and if in some instances the patient has "a right to die." "I have gotten beyond the stage concerned about technique and the notion that death implies failure," one said. People have the right to die in peace and dignity." Another explained, "The extraordinary efforts to keep some patients functioning are seen by such doctors as 'just so much medical pyrotechnics,' designed to fulfill the physician's own needs rather than those of the patient and the family." "The function of medical heroics is to demonstrate how good we are with our fancy gadgets," one said. "A good doctor can win recognition by keeping the poor old body going forever."

Physicians at this stage generally have overcome their "God complex" and recognize that physicians can, at best, only temporarily delay death.

Stage 5: Dealing With Personal Feelings

Everyone expects a good doctor to be calm, in control of his or her feelings, someone the family can rely on for support and understanding. Physicians who are anxious or fearful in the face of death must carefully conceal these emotions. "I've had a lot of training in putting up a good front so others can't see what I'm feeling inside," one said. "I've learned to keep this cool facade of being in control. But inside, I'm feeling a lot of stress."

> A nurse told me that when a patient died who had been on the floor for a long time, she decided to organize a service so that the other nurses could share their feelings. But no one showed up. One nurse said she didn't go because, "I would start to cry about all the patients I've seen die, I would never stop."

My interviews with seasoned physicians found that most of them have unresolved problems with regard to death that create severe anxieties; many wept when interviewed.[40] Remarkably, it was often the first time they had been asked about how they felt or discussed their disquieting experiences of inadvertently "killing" a patient through error or bad advice. Although technical procedures had been critically reviewed in M&M conferences, their feelings were never addressed.

Until physicians reach this stage of self-examination, they usually cope with impending death by avoidance. "I try to keep away from patients if I know what's coming up so it will reduce the emotional stress," a medical student confessed. Feelings of helplessness can be relieved by passing these patients off to someone else or by being too busy to spend a lot of time with them. The physician can simply check the equipment, write the orders, and then bustle out of the room. "We ignore the patient because we are so fearful ourselves," one acknowledged.

Typically, every effort is made in hospital settings to shield clinicians from mourning relatives. Crying is tolerated in the emergency room, but if any kind of emotional outburst occurs, relatives may be hustled off to the chapel. "We isolate them so that their grief is not so obvious," a physician said. "It isn't done cruelly, but frankly it is done more to protect the emergency room staff than to help the family."

Physicians fault their mentors in the early training years for giving them such little support when patients die. "It's almost as though I've had to deal with this part of medical practice without any preparation," one said. "In most every other aspect of my training, I've had a chance to observe my preceptors and then discuss the experience." The few who did receive instruction about death characterize it as intellectualized and abstract. It was presented, "in cookbooklike fashion, no different than if we were learning to work up a case of hypertension." "We were never asked to discuss how we felt about death." None of those interviewed could recall a single experience when clinical mentors revealed their own feelings about death—the frustrations, anger, hopelessness that occur when they lose a patient.

By examining their inner lives and identifying their feelings, doctors at this stage can become more "compleat." "I can speak for myself and possibly for a lot of other physicians," one said:

> In my younger years, my professional self-image wouldn't permit me to be slowed down or have my efficiency reduced by my feelings. So, I've been conditioned in what I now call "Disembodied Intelligence." But now I'm beginning to get more and more in touch with my own feelings, to recognize and tolerate them. It's helped me become a better physician and I try to help others work with their feelings.

Thomas McCormick, who teaches death education at the University of Washington School of Medicine, says, "A great wall of silence exists between physicians and their patients in talking about death." He believes that teaching medical students how to communicate better with their dying patients can break down that wall.[41] At some schools, students are taught how to help the family when a loved one dies:

> I was in a small group that discussed how to deliver bad news and deal with cancer and dying. One physician told us that no matter how busy you or the hospital staff are, when someone dies, always provide time for the family to be with the deceased patient. If the death occurs in the ER, place the patient on a regular bed and cover up any disfigurement. Also, place the patient's hand outside the bedsheet because the family will always want to hold it. You have to let them say good-bye.

Some medical schools have recently instituted thanatology education. Students have interaction with a terminally ill patient, either through direct involvement or observation of patient-physician interactions. Small group discussions where students talk about their own feelings regarding death and dying are an integral aspect of these courses. Also discussed are such ethically complicated topics as living wills, advanced directives, surrogate makers, euthanasia, and physician-assisted suicides. To help students learn more about these complex issues, the 1996 AMSA task force on death and dying established a death-and-dying resource library and compiled a curriculum guide for death-and-dying electives offered at medical schools around the country.[42]

Insights:
Responding to Difficult People
Bernard Virshup, MD

Physicians often deal with difficult people, of whom there are many—and not all of them are patients. In a larger sense, there are no difficult people, only people with whom we have difficulty dealing. All patients will be difficult for us if our sense of self requires that we heal all illness, prevent all deaths, and have everyone like and respect us.

Coping with difficult people has four aspects:

- Why are difficult people so difficult?
- Why do we react to them so?
- How do we stay centered?
- How can we cope effectively with them?

All people you see in the hospital or who come into your office have anxiety. They are anxious about their condition, about whether or not their symptoms are serious, and about the possibility of treatment. Most of these people respond well to active listening, empathic understanding, and reassurance. If, however, they meet the wall of professional distance, they are likely to become resentful and angry and, when things go wrong, bring malpractice suits. These are not truly difficult patients; they are patients made difficult by the inept physician.

Others are truly difficult for anyone to deal with. To cope effectively with these difficult people, we need to understand what makes them so difficult. A simple and useful theory is that such people are damaged; they believe that some aspect of their existence is in danger, that you not adequately protecting them or may even be responsible for their danger, and they are in the grip of excessive anxiety or even panic, which they may cover with unrealistic demands, denial, or aggressive behavior.

In his article "Taking Care of the Hateful Patient," James Groves wrote that there are three classes of patients that physicians dread most: (a) entitled demanders, (b) dependent clingers, and (c) help rejecters and deniers.[43] Entitled demanders are critical-compulsive people who have erected unrealistic standards of behavior to maintain the rigid structure of their own insecure world. If you don't do what they say, you are threatening their security. They must use coercion to get you to do what they want. They were often abused as children, and this is the only way they know to keep themselves and their world together. If you fail, they become aggressive-angry-abusive. The sense of entitlement is a pathetic sham that temporarily supports the patient's unstable psychological structure. Their anger at the physician reflects their anger at life.

Dependent clingers are needy, helpless people who need you to take care of them. All patients regress, more or less, to a childhood, Mommy-take-care-of-me state. Dependent clingers are a bottomless pit. Never having received enough love as children, they are always testing. You are a wonderful person as long as you are being a "Mommy," but it is never enough, and you must keep giving and giving until you give up giving. They often use flattery and conscious or unconscious seduction. Many of them are actually passive-aggressive people simmering with resentment and suppressed anger at a cruel and unsympathetic world (except for you, of course—as long as you keep giving of yourself).

Help rejecters and deniers are another manifestation of passive-aggressiveness. Help rejecters have inexhaustible ways to frustrate you and exhaust your patience. Help rejecters feel that no regimen will help and return again and again to report that, once again, the treatment did not help. Deniers deny infirmity, chafe under medical restrictions and continue practices that injure their own health, for example, alcoholics who drink, emphysema patients who smoke, coronary patients who continue to gorge on fats, and so on. Why do we react to them so?

We tend to believe, "He made me angry." "She got me upset." But in a larger sense, we make ourselves angry or upset or depressed by what we think about what happened. Other people do what they do. We react to it the way we react. Of his angina one man said, "My life is in the hands of any fool who chooses to make me angry." And, indeed, he died of his coronary artery disease in an apoplectic fit of anger. But who was really the "fool"?

So, how do we upset ourselves? The main way is to believe that our sense of self-worth is somehow being threatened. Our conditional sense of self is evoked by difficult people.

Entitled demanders tell us we're not measuring up to their standards. We all carry a small internal critic that concurs that we are incompetent, inadequate, disorganized, stupid, and ineffective and that we should shape up to amount to anything. Entitled demanders hook into our own internal critic by using intimidation, criticism, devaluation, and guilt. They bully us by invoking painful shadows of past episodes of rejection, humiliation, irresponsibility, and shame. We may regress to childhood reactions of appeasement or anger. We may "dexify"—try to defend, explain and justify—so that the angry person will stop being angry with us.

Needy, helpless, bottomless pit dependent clingers take advantage of our genuine wish to do good—a wish that may have contributed to our being in a helping profession in the first place—and our guilt if we turn away.

Passive-aggressive help rejecters and deniers drive us crazy by rejecting our help and in effect making us ineffectual. We react most often by getting angry at them for "wasting our time. If they're not going to take our advice, why are they coming here?" And they make us doubt ourselves and feel inadequate.

To cope with difficult people, we must learn to remain centered. That has to do with our unconditional sense of self, with our ability to say to ourselves,

"I am a good, competent, caring person." "I do what I do because I am a good, competent, caring person." "I don't have to do anything to prove it."

Coping with these difficult people requires three steps: (a) active listening is essential ("I hear and understand what you want of me, and why you want it"); (b) self-centering is most important (silently saying to yourself, "I know I'm all right, and I don't have to prove it"); and (c) you must take responsibility for doing and saying what you think is best ("This is what I'm willing to do"), rather then merely reacting. If we can truly stay centered, we can accept our real and practical responsibilities and limits, which includes taking care of others' needs with due consideration for our own, without feeling selfish, rude, or somehow wrong or inadequate. The end result will be that we will be assertive and creative. We are, in effect, saying to others, "I respect you, and what you need to do for yourself; and I respect myself and what I have to do just as much." Instead of reacting with anger, deprecation, or defensiveness, we can substitute for the "broken record" by affirming the other's position and then affirming our own.

Difficult people frustrate our need to feel good about ourselves; they make us insecure and doubtful of our own worth. If our self-worth is secure, we can look at the difficult person and ask, "What's that about? What's going on?" If we aren't defensive or judgmental but genuinely interested, we are likely to hear some story of unfilled psychological needs. We can then make decisions as to how much we are willing to do to satisfy those needs and our own.

Notes

1. Hilfiker, David. 1986. "Facing Our Mistakes." In Robert H. Coombs, D. Scott May, and Gary W. Small, eds. *Inside Doctoring: Stages and Outcomes in the Professional Development of Physicians* (pp. 163-171). New York: Praeger, p. 169.

2. "Hospital Errors." 1995, August. *Health Letter* (Public Citizens Health Research Group, Dr. Sidney M. Wolfe, ed.), 11(8):5-7, 11, p. 5. [This report was excerpted from an ABC "Nightline" program aired July 4, 1995]

3. *Ibid.*

4. *Ibid.*, pp. 6-7.

5. Hilfiker, *op. cit.*

6. *Ibid.*, p. 169.

7. Alessio, Carolyn. 1997, January-February. "Trial and Error." *The New Physician*, pp. 47-48, p. 48.

8. Koelbl, James J. 1991. "Patients With AIDS: Do We Have a Duty To Treat? Part 1." *The Compendium*, 12(9):676, 678, 680.

9. Rosenthal, Elisabeth. 1989, September. "Coming of Age With AIDS." *Discover,* 34:36-37, p. 36.

10. Currey, Charles J., Michael Johnson, and Barbara Ogden. 1990. "Willingness of Health-Professions Students to Treat Patients with AIDS." *Academic Medicine,* 65(7):472-474.

11. Rosenthal, *op. cit.,* p. 36.

12. Turk, Michele. 1993, September. "High Anxiety." *The New Physician,* pp. 16-22.

13. *Ibid.*

14. *Ibid.,* p. 20.

15. *Ibid.,* p. 19.

16. *Ibid,,* p. 20.

17. Boyd, Susan J. 1996, March. "Needlestick." *The New Physician,* pp. 35-36, p. 35.

18. *Ibid,* pp. 35-36.

19. Turk, *op. cit.*

20. Koelbl, *op. cit.,* p. 680.

21. Magaro, Amy. 1993, September. "The Medical Expertise Retention Program (MERP)." *The New Physician,* p. 21.

22. Shorr, Andrew F. 1995, Spring. "Health Care Workers, Patients, and HIV: An Analysis of the Policy and Ethical Debate." *The Pharos,* pp. 7-13.

23. Monmaney, Terence. 1996, February 29. "Doctor Gave Hepatitis to 19 Patients at UCLA." *Los Angeles Times,* pp. B1, B6.

24. Greengard, Samuel. 1991, October 21. "Problem Patients." *American Medical News,* pp. 21-22, p. 22.

25. *Ibid.*

26. *Ibid.*

27. *Ibid.,* pp. 21-22.

28. *Ibid.,* p. 22.

29. *Ibid.*

30. *Ibid.*

31. Coombs, Robert H., Sangeeta Chopra, Debra Schenk, and Elaine Yutan. 1993. "Medical Slang and Its Functions." *Social Science and Medicine,* 36(8):987-998, p. 996.

32. Coombs, Robert H., and Linda J. Goldman. 1973. "Maintenance and Discontinuity of Coping Mechanisms in an Intensive Care Unit." *Social Problems,* 20(3):342-352.

33. Coombs, Chopra, Schenk, and Yutan, *op. cit.,* p. 987.

34. Orwell, George. 1954. *A Collection of Essays.* Garden City, NY: Doublesday, p. 173.

35. Coombs, Chopra, Schenk, and Yutan, *op. cit.,* p. 996.

36. *Ibid.*

37. Finkelstein, Peter. 1986. "Studies in the Anatomy Laboratory: A Portrait of Individual and Collective Defense." In Robert H. Coombs, D. Scott May, and Gary W. Small, eds. *Inside Doctoring: Stages and Outcomes in the Professional Development of Physicians* (pp. 22-42). New York: Praeger.

38. Lief, Harold I., and Renee C. Fox C. 1963. "Training for 'Detached Concern' in Medical Students." In Harold I. Lief, V. Lief, and N. R. Lief, eds. *The Psychological Basis of Medical Practice* (pp. 12-35). New York: Hoeber Medical Division, Harper & Row.

39. Coombs, Robert H., and Pauline S. Powers. 1975, October. "Socialization for Death." *Urban Life,* pp. 251-271.

40. *Ibid.*

41. Rutter, Terry. 1996, March. "Spotlight: Mortality and Medical Education." *The New Physician,* p. 6.

42. *Ibid.*

43. Groves, James E. 1978. "Taking Care of the Hateful Patient." *New England Journal of Medicine,* 298(16):883-887.

CHAPTER 8

Fourth Year

Will I Ever Know Enough?

*During the internship I'm going to find out essentially how competent
I am. Right now I'm still in the dark about my ability.*

—Fourth-year medical student

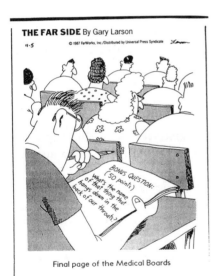

THE FAR SIDE By Gary Larson
11-5 © 1987 FarWorks, Inc./Distributed by Universal Press Syndicate

BONUS QUESTION:
(50 points)
What's the name
of that thing that
hangs down in the
back of our throats?

Final page of the Medical Boards

Some fourth-year medical students contend they haven't really changed, just matured. Others are more aware of altered perceptions and attitudes—toward themselves, their peers, "the system," and, in particular, their medical careers. In short, they "look at things differently now." "One thing for sure," a fourth-year student remarked, "you do get the MD degree after a four-year grueling, frustrating, and fascinating process."

Senior Metamorphosis

Seniors talk about being "toned down, less wild." Coupled with this increased seriousness is a new conservatism, both social and political. Some fourth-year students are surprised to find themselves suddenly understanding and even agreeing with parental attitudes they rejected a few years before. They describe themselves as being more "realistic" or "practical," meaning they are now less willing to take personal and professional risks. They are not about to throw away three difficult years of training by "rocking the boat." The shift from idealism to greater practicality may be seen as "increasing selfishness" or part of a logical growth process in which medicine represents a "job much like any other": "We'll be serving the needs of the public, but we'll also be providing for our own families."

As a senior facing the increased independence and responsibility of internship, you may well take satisfaction in "learning to think for yourself and knowing yourself, your weaknesses and strengths, a whole lot better than when you entered med school." And you may find "your intellectual capacity is markedly increased. You're able to comprehend more complex and lengthier materials in a shorter span of time." You may even find yourself becoming like some fourth-year students who are "kind of headstrong or conceited." One fact is certain: The changes are irreversible.

Self-Concept

Having survived the first three years of medical school and being within sight of a long-cherished goal gives most seniors a sense of accomplishment and a good measure of self-confidence.

"It sneaks up on you. You sort of shut your eyes and do all your work, and then in a month or two you look back and realize you're a bit closer than you were." "Most of us enjoy being at least competent. They treat us more like doctors now." Some explain their heightened sense of self-worth in terms of service: "The modest success I've had helping patients boosts my self-image a little. It's good knowing you're in a position where you could probably help people on your own, without guidance from somebody."

Fourth-year students find themselves able to adapt quickly to different situations. "I don't think there's any great revelation. It's just practice, continuous practice." "You handle a few situations competently and you become so proud. You think, 'Maybe I *am* a good doctor.'"

You'll likely feel an intensified need to learn, not just to pass exams, not just to get by on the floor without looking foolish, but to be equipped for the challenges that are very near. "One way to think of yourself as a doctor is by wearing a white coat; the other way is by becoming proficient in the skills you must develop."

Relations With Peers and Family

By the senior year, the regional and ethnic differences between class-mates, so apparent to first- and second-year students, blur or disappear:

> The first two years in the classroom, Chicanos sat with Chicanos, blacks with blacks, Iranians with Iranians, boisterous personalities with boister-ous personalities, Southerners with Southerners, and so on. Now we're all randomly selected into different groups and just thrown into the ring with one another. The blending has been a good experience.

> Moving closer to graduation, stereotypes and distinctions between stu-dents (North/South, ethnic, religious, common outside interests) don't really disappear but change to specialty interest and career aspirations. Surgeons are the class "gunners," medicine hopefuls like to think about differential diagnoses, dermatology and radiology hopefuls think about vacation possibilities.

Fourth-year medical students, scattered about in different clinical rota-tions throughout the university hospital and community, rarely, if ever, come together as a class. "During the clinical years you only have contact with one to four classmates at a time, so social contacts are difficult." Some feel the arrangement broadens their perspectives and brings individuals closer to-gether:

> Clinical rotations allowed me to get to know and become friends with classmates that I probably wouldn't have sought out otherwise. You find yourself eager to share your experiences and give pointers on what to do and what not to do, which residents to avoid. You feel for them, especially classmates who are on a brutal rotation that you've already been through.

When you do see each other you will continue to assist one another informally by sharing interesting patients and clinical problems: "There's a freer ex-change of knowledge—and lack of knowledge—this year." Some students estimate that aside from their reading 50% to 60% of what they learn comes from the house staff and the rest from fellow students and clinical faculty. "When I come up with a problem and another student sits down and takes the time to explain and teach me something, that's just about the best thing any-body could do for me." "A lot of people are finding their own niches that they like and have been reading about. They know a lot more in that area than anybody else and you can pick up little pearls from them." "As a fourth-year, I find that third-year students ask me a lot of questions, and I like to teach."

Fourth-year students discover new respect for their classmates: "I've been surprised to see that some of those I thought in the first two years wouldn't make good doctors have really come into their own on clinical services and will probably be good physicians." "Some of these people I really enjoy working with. They carry their own load, have a good relationship with patients, and the patients seem to like them."

A few students at this stage are indifferent or even antagonistic toward classmates: "I'm very embittered this year. They haven't done anything for me. There are very few I would care to see again after I graduate, and I won't be crushed if I don't see them at all." More likely, however, you will feel a bit wrenched by separation from your comrades after graduation:

> Because of the *intense* social and emotional relationships that develop between students—some of the most meaningful experiences I've ever had—I dread the day when everyone in the class will be scattered around the country. The stress of seeing these relationships end in the fourth year is as severe as any trauma in med school—even a pathology exam.

You may also be surprised by developments in your relationships with your family and friends: "I'm beginning to realize I'm going to be separated from my family more than I thought. Which is going to come first? What I thought was going to work out probably isn't." "I have different relationships now than I did before med school." "You talk about medicine quite a lot when you go home. You don't realize how much of your existence is medically oriented and that you really don't know what's going on in the outside world. You sort of lose touch with that reality." "In terms of social and ethical progress, I don't think medicine does anything for you." "It's easy to get apathetic about things not related to medicine."

Accepting the System

Although some fourth-year students still regard basic science instruction as "oriented toward graduate students and not doctors-to-be, totally useless for what we have to do," for the most part you will cease to devote energy to changing the system or even complaining about it. Some seniors acknowledge that they have no real notion, despite their early outrage, of what significant change could be introduced into the first two years "where most of the stress is."

You may be one of the students who continue to think of PhD science instructors as having been "cooped up in their labs a little too long," and you may wish they could be "taken out on a ward and shown where all their molecules and chemicals really fit in—not in a test tube, but in a human being," but the chances are good that you'll say, "Looking back, I don't dislike the first two years as much as I thought I did. In fact, I sort of liked them."

By your fourth year, you will probably have revised your perception of just what "the system" is all about. Most seniors do. They're less sure than lower-division students that the system *should* be "beaten": "The only thing you can beat now is yourself by not getting the education you're here for." "When you're part of the system, it's hard to beat it." "The only way to beat the system is to play the rules of the game." One even admitted, "I'm not even sure anymore what 'the system' is—maybe just to graduate!"

A great sense of impending responsibility makes most seniors eager to learn from house staff and clinical faculty. Fourth-year students are appreciative of the time taken with them, the patience shown, and especially of the generally kind way in which their mistakes are treated—although "mistakes are treated much more kindly during the third year than the fourth! As a fourth year, one is 'supposed to know better.'" Fourth-year students particularly appreciate house staff who take extra time to explain and teach individually. Whether they perceive faculty and staff members' interest in them as "parental," as an attempt to welcome neophytes "into the circle," as a desire to have the school well represented by its interns, or as a self-serving "attempt to curry favor and attract some interns," most seniors are grateful for it. Seniors respond by making a conscious effort to build good feelings and to minimize potential friction, acting in an "appropriate" manner by going out of their way to be interested, to be available, to do particularly thorough work-ups, and to avoid giving the impression of being a "wiseass."

Many seniors happily note a more cooperative and respectful attitude from the nursing staff than they experienced as juniors. Some mention coming back after semester break and being treated as if they had a new "aura" that made them more acceptable. Others explain the change in terms of their own greater experience, confidence, and tact in working with nurses and other hospital personnel. This shift in others' attitudes toward you will be one of the most important developments of your senior year. Status recognition by professional peers is one of the surest ways young physicians begin to accept their new roles as doctors.

Probably the most dramatic difference between first- and fourth-year medical students is their perception of the medical profession. A fourth-year student reflected,

> You become more disciplined and therefore a little more conservative, more practical and less idealistic; and this all happens so fast, in just four years. You're aware of what's happening, and you sort of get disgusted with yourself at times that you're allowing yourself to be molded. And yet some of the old ideals and thoughts are still there.

A fellow, who as an undergraduate took a course on the psychosocial dynamics of medical school, observed,

> I anticipated that I'd experience a lot of personal sacrifices and would never feel comfortable at the hospital, never find meaningful friendships amongst other physicians—constant fighting in a stifling political atmosphere. But I persisted in my career goals because I wanted to take care of patients and experience the academic and ethical challenges of medicine. Now that I've gone through the hardest part, I'm pleased to say I do feel fine in a hospital setting. I feel like part of a team that works and sometimes even plays well together. Some of my best friends are physicians. They are some of the most interesting people I've ever met. There are as many radicals and liberals and goofy doctors as laypersons in the community at large. And, it is strange, but I find myself frequently rising to the defense of this medical establishment.

Seniors differ from lower-division students in another important respect. No longer forced to "book it" every waking hour, they are nonetheless totally committed to their work. Only now, the commitment isn't to medical school, but to medicine.

Emotional Distancing From Patients

By now, you will have learned to maintain emotional distance from patients. You may call this cynicism or a survival mechanism or consider it necessary to maintain scientific objectivity for optimum patient care. This change is a definite by-product of your medical education, albeit one that is not formally taught:

Earlier in the clinical experience, I identified more with patients, taking what they say at face value, being on their side. But I find myself gradually shifting, becoming more skeptical, more discriminating when I hear patient complaints. I'm inching closer to the house staff perspective.

As a senior, you may be unsure of the significance of this change in yourself and even defensive about it: "The only way I can see to cope is dissociation and desensitization." "I think you become detached, rather than dehumanized. I try to appear more cynical than I really am." "I'm just the opposite; I've become more sensitive to problems. Still, I must build a wall to keep from being affected by every bit of suffering." And, although you may be concerned about your diminished sensitivity, you'll certainly agree that "You can't die with every patient."

You may even attribute at least a part of your new emotional distance to your patients, from whom you are "constantly hearing complaints about conditions with no actual organic basis." "Such patients," one said, "can lead students and doctors to become cynical." "A freshman would interview a patient and come out saying, 'Boy, that's really a sad story. He's really sick and has a lot of problems.' A senior seeing the same patient would say, 'Damn crock! What's he here for? Why doesn't he see a psychiatrist?'"

Acceptance of Physician Fallibility

Fourth-year students have learned that no physician provides perfect, error-free diagnosis and treatment:

You become a little more skeptical about what medicine can do for people. At first I thought medicine could cure almost anything, diagnose almost everything, help anybody. As you go on, you find there are a lot of diseases doctors never diagnose and patients they are never able to help.

"You realize you aren't God. You can't do all things, be all things, for all people."

Once you accept the reality of medical fallibility, you can acknowledge that some mistakes may be your own. Sleep deprivation no doubt contributes to this risk.[1] You may realize that a mistake may eventually cost a patient's life: "I haven't made any big mistakes yet—no lives have been lost because of me. The first time I lose a patient because of my mistakes I'm going to be upset about it."

Students prepare themselves for this harsh reality: "I'll try to rationalize it." "Everybody makes mistakes. But you try not to make the same one twice."

> You resign yourself to the fact that you're not perfect. Most people who go into medicine are kind of egotistical and like to think they are perfect, but they get knocked down and beaten during medical school and begin to realize there's nothing to be done about it; they're going to make mistakes.

You will probably experience a loss of idealism as a senior, a result of experiencing the medical system at work. Although some students argue that "patients receive outstanding care from interns and residents," others are less sanguine:

> Sure, you tend to become cynical. As a student you work with a lot of clinic patients who can't afford a private doctor, so they're the guinea pigs of the hospital at the disposal of the interns and residents as part of their training. You do see some gross negligence, and you see patients paying outlandish prices for diagnostic procedures that are part of the training program—done for teaching purposes rather than for the patients.

You also may resent the demands on you and staff members that preclude giving personalized care to patients. The cost of health care and the absence of adequate health plans may also prove disturbing: "I've seen too many cases of people not coming to the hospital because they couldn't afford it and letting their diseases get out of hand because they didn't have the money to pay the hospital bill." Note this student's struggle to maintain idealism:

> Although I didn't come in with the idea that all MDs knew what they were doing, I felt that, by God, I was going to be an excellent MD, compassionate, caring for the patients, valuing their opinions, and an expert in my field. I didn't believe them when they told me that slowly over time I would relate less and less to patients and begin to empathize more and more with the MD. But it did occur to some extent, and although I try desperately not to show it, there are times when I feel less compassionate than I used to. I have the long hours and abusive treatment of medical

students during the clinical years to thank for that. It is important that students realize this is an "O.K." human reaction to the working conditions and to constantly make it a top priority to treat all patients with the dignity and respect that they deserve. That doesn't mean you have to always feel empathetic, etc., so long as you do what is best for the patients—both medically and emotionally.

Part of the emotional distancing you develop on the clinical floors will affect your personal life: "When I hear that a friend is sick or when one of my wife's friends miscarries, it really doesn't bother me at all. I've seen it happen to so many people, it's hard for me to imagine *anybody* being well." "I find that as soon as someone starts to discuss a medical problem, questions fill my mind. I can no longer be just an involved and supportive listener. I have to analyze the problem clinically!" "My folks think I've been terribly cynical. My mother doesn't like it, but my uncle, who's a doctor, doesn't seem to mind."

Just as experience blunts sensitivity to suffering and hopes of infallibility, so idealism can be badly shaken by the real world of clinical practice:

> I used to think of being a missionary. Now, in the clinic, I see more and more lower-class people. I was never exposed to them before, and I'm beginning to realize that I don't relate well to these people. I feel kind of uncomfortable. I still feel sorry for them, but somehow I've begun to enjoy my work more when I'm with middle-class people. Doctors go live in the middle-class communities, and then the lower classes get no doctors. It's too bad.

"You start out gung ho, wanting to work for nothing and save the world. As a senior, you're more interested in money and getting a salary instead of paying tuition."

External Rewards

The "service to humanity" theme that runs through the conversations of entering first-year students is far less prevalent among seniors, whereas the "economic security" motif, of only passing interest to first-year students, assumes major importance for seniors. Many medical students graduate with a large debt that must be serviced during their residency, forcing them to moonlight or enter medical practice immediately after residency:[2] "I've got to pay back a hundred Gs in loans!" Only a few students can say, "I don't owe any-body anything for my education. My MD is mine and my wife's and nobody else's. Nobody helped us. It's a very proud feeling."

Most seniors, now in their late 20s or early 30s, have never been finan-cially independent, and many still face years of economic strain and continu-ing indebtedness. It is understandable that many define their career aspira-tions in terms of income: "Doctors make good money." "Medicine has all the attributes that would make somebody go into it. It's financially rewarding and it's got a bit of luster to it." "I went into medicine because it was lucrative." "The financial reward is better than average." Entering first-year students tend to view their future careers in terms of serving their fellow human be-ings, contributing to the world's knowledge, and participating in scientific breakthroughs; seniors are much more attuned to tangible rewards. Four years of hard work, ego battering, and financial deprivation, coupled with new so-phistication about the realities of medicine, dramatically color their thinking. Most still welcome the idea of helping people, but few seniors focus solely on that goal.

Seniors are more willing and able than lower-division students to specu-late on the income they hope to realize as physicians. They are also more attuned to the social status doctors enjoy and look forward to a time when they will not be "just students" but respected and productive members of the com-munity. Both financial rewards and social recognition become important mo-tivators for practicing medicine. "After what we've been through, I can con-fidently say we deserve it!" These rewards, however, have become less certain. Even the respect traditionally accorded the physician has been eroded somewhat by a more cynical view of doctors as greedy and exploitative: "Doctors no longer retain as high societal position. Financial stability is now uncertain, though we know we'll live comfortably."

Another motivating factor once cited by medical students is disappear-ing—the concept of the physician as his or her own boss. Medical graduates who launch into private practice are likely to join established practices as junior members. Still more common today is going to work for a health main-tenance organization (HMO).

The desire for prestige, appreciative patients, financial security, and in-dependence is intense and understandable in the fourth year. For most of you, these desires will be combined with a strong positive conviction about your future career. "I have absolutely no regrets about going into medicine. I think it's possible to do great things, help people a lot. As for my own aspirations, being creative and developing a sense of self-confidence and prestige, it's great!" But in the fourth year, the rewards, the prestige, and the security are still a dream far off and a giant step away—after residency training.

Handling Doubts

Some of the confidence you gain from your clinical experience will melt with the prospect of soloing as an intern or resident. You're likely to think, "I need a resident around. I'm not ready to go out and practice medicine." You can no longer say, "I don't know," and then refer the patient to a resident while you go away to look up answers. You'll soon have to respond to questions and emergencies with your own knowledge and experience. As a resident, you'll be directly on the firing line, required to know and do on the spot. For most fourth-year students, this is an awesome prospect. "As internship approaches, I find myself studying and reviewing during my time off. I dread making a mistake that may adversely affect someone's life. I don't know how much the reviewing will help, but it relieves some of the anxiety."

If your clinical approach as a student is more style than substance, dealing with patients by "acting in a professional and dignified manner, not showing any weakness," you may become acutely aware of your shortcomings when you face the challenge of actually taking charge.

How do you deal with your own insecurity when treating patients? First, "become confident in the ability to do the procedure, just be competent." "I try to be sure what I'm doing before I see the patient, and I try not to display any anxiety when I go in." Some contend that patients will tolerate uncertainty if it is presented honestly: "Patients lose confidence in you not so much because you can't do a procedure but because you won't admit you can't do it." Some students concentrate on cultivating techniques of effective communication, "developing rapport with a patient, offering reassurance, spending time with him." "Take a minute to stop and talk." "Try not to be dogmatic. Take time to listen to complaints." By the end of your fourth year, your bedside manner had better be backed up with some solid skills, because when you enter your residency you'll need a real sense of "ease with your own abilities."

Some students expect their doubts and insecurities to vanish automatically when there is no one else to make decisions: "I'll run out of bucks to pass, and then I'll have to take responsibility." "After I do it for a little while, I think I'll have confidence." Others recognize that it's probably overly optimistic to expect a sudden change in their perception of their own abilities: "kind of hope that somebody will touch me with a wand on graduation day." Other students are pessimistic: "I feel like I'm going in reverse—learning a little less every day. By the end, I feel I'll know nothing." "The point has been driven home how little I know. I missed a couple of cases of measles this year—and there are a lot of other disease entities to miss."

Fourth-year students recognize how protected they have been and that this protection is about to disappear. They have no real basis for determining whether their knowledge and abilities are adequate:

> You have to try before you know. Now, how many times have I had the chance to try an independent diagnosis? We have a patient come in and you have to hold your hands over your ears to keep somebody—even the patient—from telling you that "Dr. So-and-So says I've got such-and-such."

"We're in an ivory tower over here. It's probably going to be a rude shock when we leave. We're seeing a very narrow segment of medicine." A few fourth-year students see a positive side to their self-doubting: "It's important for you to realize you're not going to know it all. You have to make an effort to continue your education."

It may be consoling to recognize that you are not alone in your fears and feelings of inadequacy. "Here we are, future doctors, and I realize we aren't the perfect beings we thought we were going to be." "I talk to the people I hang out with, wondering if we're really prepared for internship. It seems to be the thing most of us worry about more than anything else." "I don't think I'm less competent than the rest of my classmates, but I just wonder how competent any of us are."

But for all the self-doubts and fears, most fourth-year students are still eager to take the next step in their learning process. "You have to try before you know. I think I'm ready to try." Typically, they believe—and hope—they will become competent physicians through a gradual process, details of which aren't yet perceptible to them: "After all, I'm still a fourth-year student. I'm not competent yet to do the work of a doctor who's been in practice for 20 years." "It helps to compare myself as a graduating fourth-year student to the new interns I remember seeing at the beginning of this year. I don't think our level of knowledge is that much different. If they made it, I know I will, too." "Of course, I'm not confident. That's the reason for internship."

What Makes a Good Doctor?

By the end of your clinical clerkships, you will most likely have formed a fairly strong idea of the qualities possessed by good doctors and what characteristics are typical of inferior ones. This assessment will reflect your own values and the physicians you've observed. In some ways, it will also reflect your own preferences concerning the area of medicine in which you'd like to practice.

Some students define good doctors according to the way they practice:

There are two kinds of good doctors. In the medical center, it's somebody who knows as much as humanly possible about a specific field and who keeps in mind the concept of the total patient. She doesn't treat a liver, but a patient with liver disease. The community doctor has factual knowledge, but not necessarily as much as the one in the academic setting. She has a concept of her patient as a human being and also keeps in mind the patient's position in his family, community, and day-to-day life. For example, if she could possibly avoid it, a good doctor wouldn't take a man who's always been a dynamic go-getter and put him on bed rest, because it would ruin the guy.

Another concept of the good doctor is that he or she is simply "a good person." "A good doctor has many of the same qualities as a good lawyer, a good teacher, or a good housewife." A good doctor is "competent, knows his limitations." He "enjoys good relations with patients and does the best he can for them." She's "satisfied that she's doing a good job. If this is merely talking to a crock once a week and letting him get everything off his chest, then that's a good doctor." A good doctor "has time to listen to patients' problems, is technically and emotionally stable, and is intelligent." She is "knowledgeable but humble, confident, and knows her limits." A good doctor "doesn't get frustrated easily," is "current in his field, up-to-date," and can "adapt to any kind of patient personality." A good doctor's approach to patients is "firm, but gentle."

The closer I get to residency, the more concerned I am about remembering everything. Fourth-year electives are often specialized and I feel myself forgetting many vital things I learned the last two years and knew well at one point. That's distressing. Another concern is integrating personality traits of a good physician with the factual knowledge of a good physician. I find myself falling back on role models I have worked with. In school, we demonstrate interpersonal skills in our interaction with patients and demonstrate factual knowledge in our interaction with residents and attendings. Rarely do we as students see patients, do the history and physical, then discuss diagnostic possibilities, a proposed plan of action and treatment possibilities with pros and cons of options without first discussing the case with an attending or resident.

By their fourth year in medical school, many students see intellectual capacity as counting less than honesty and attentiveness to the patient: "I find myself much more critical and less tolerant about deficits in a physician's knowledge-base when he has poor interpersonal skills. I'm much more forgiving toward physicians who are good 'people persons.'" A good doctor, "even though she might not have quite as much knowledge, has common sense, and is hardworking enough so that when she sees a patient she doesn't just brush by. She thinks about the patient." Compassion is important, and so is patience. A good doctor is able to organize what the patient is saying into a relevant body of information that leads to an accurate diagnosis. Concomitant with acknowledging and accepting fallibility is the desire among fourth-year students to remain sensitive to problems they can't and shouldn't attempt to handle. They ascribe to good doctors "sufficient confidence to diagnose and treat certain problems and refer other problems to somebody else."

Interestingly, in terms of their own self-doubts in the face of medical practice, many students see the absence of self-assurance as one characteristic of a bad doctor: "Good intentions and competence are not enough. If the student doesn't have confidence in his or her medical knowledge, that person certainly is not going to become a good doctor."

Most students define bad doctors with reference more to their lack of concern with patients and their basic arrogance than to dearth of medical skills:

By and large, you find you will be forgiven for ignorance or making a mistake (if it's not too bad); what will ruin you is if, for example, you lie. Somebody got thrown out of my medical school for making a rude remark to a woman patient during her pelvic exam. Issues of behavior and personal conduct are in fact mentioned during "the cramming years," but you'd never believe how they end up outweighing all the science minutiae you learn and forget.

No matter how outstanding a doctor's technical abilities, one who "doesn't treat the patient as a person" is not practicing good medicine. Some students think a bad doctor exhibits these traits because of "a dislike for the work—a feeling of being in the wrong business." And some students see that the designation of a bad doctor may depend largely on the point of view of the observer: "In the eyes of a physician, it's somebody not capable of administering good patient care. For the patients' families and the rest of our society, a bad doctor is some one who cannot relate to them as people." "If doctors continue to act arrogant, aloof, and humorless, if they continue to act like cold fish," one physician noted, "the malpractice lawyers will eat them like sushi."[3]

Specialization: Looking Ahead

As a senior, you'll probably be very sensitive to the enormity of the decisions you face, and you'll feel tremendous pressure. Part of the pressure will be to secure a good residency that will enhance your education and carry with it some prestige. Another source of pressure may be your family and financial situation. A prolonged period of residency and the further possibility of a fellowship extends the duration of financial dependency. The more complex the specialty or subspecialty you choose, the longer you defer any financial return and the greater is the sacrifice by those who are dependent on you or on whom you depend. This knowledge adds to the stresses of choosing the "right" specialty immediately and not wasting time shopping around. In fact, as early as halfway through your third year you may be expected to begin focusing on a specialty.

Specialty Choice

Some students decide on their specialty before entering medical school, but most vacillate, particularly after some clinical experience: "I had the problem of enjoying every service I rotated through. I wish I had liked one best. I'd be better equipped to decide." "I've changed about four times between neurology and medicine."

Perhaps, you'll be one of the lucky few for whom career choice is no problem: "I know what I want to do and where I want to intern." "I've always wanted to be a psychiatrist." More likely, you'll be among the majority who choose a specialty as a result of direct experience on the clinical floors, through contact with some particularly impressive individuals, or possibly even because of family influence: "After experiencing different fields, you may find one that has the greatest interest and gives the most personal satisfaction. It's the service you go back to on off-duty hours, the one you can spend time on when you don't have to be there." "You find something you feel comfortable with. It's exciting to you." Others use a negative process: "It's a matter of exclusion, mainly excluding things you dislike."

Some seniors, unsure at the time of graduation, hope to gain clearer direction during residency. A quarter of all medical students change their specialty choice after graduation, sometimes after unhappy years practicing in an unrewarding field.[4] As graduation approaches, most fourth-year students keenly feel the need to make some commitment, not only because of the immediacy of residency, but also because they are reluctant to lose any more time or money.

There are so many factors to consider in selecting a specialty and applying for a residency, you will probably find the decision an agonizing one. What are the latest trends in the marketplace? There may be a glut in one field—radiology, for example—where incomes plummeted. Who could have predicted the growth of HMOs, PPOs (preferred provider organizations), IPAs (independent physician associations) a short time ago or the increased demand for primary care practitioners? "It's a big decision and can cause stress. A lot of people are forced into making a decision—at least a basic decision between a medical and surgical residency—earlier than they would like." "Many of my classmates lament the fact that we had to apply for residency before completing the core classes. Many times, we make career decisions on blind faith alone." "You have the feeling that you're making a life career choice before you're ready. You're determining the rest of your life."

Chances are, however, that by your fourth year you will have strong opinions, even if you aren't absolutely ready to decide. And, like your classmates, you may stereotype practitioners of various specialties—neurologists as brainy, psychiatrists as crazy, pathologists as ghoulish, dermatologists as superficial, and so on—and use slang terms to describe them. Typically, you'll regard your own specialty choice as best, one that attracts people of outstanding merit and admirable traits. You'll probably assign your own preference near the top of the status ladder.

You may adopt slang terms to poke fun at specialists. For example, surgeons may be called "blades" or "sturgeons"; orthopedists, "bones," "bone bangers," "bone crushers," "pods," or "orthopods"; urologists, "dick docs," "stream team," or "piss prophets"; gynecologists, "gyneguys" or "gynetrons"; obstetricians, "baby catchers," "crotch docs," or "placenta helpers"; otolaryngologists, "booger pickers"; anesthesiologists, "gas passers"; psychiatrists, "spooks" or "psychlotrons"; neurologists, "neurons"; pediatricians, "pedipods" or "veterinarians"; pathologists, "scope jockeys"; and dentists "tooth fairies."

How you choose will have a lot to do with your personal style. You may narrow down your options by judging how much time you want to give, what's most compatible with the lifestyle you want, the level of personal contact you want with patients, the degree of follow-up you want, how much money you plan to make, what kind of social prestige you want, and even what your spouse thinks.

> The best advice I received on choosing a field was from an instructor who told me, "First, you have to sit down and be totally honest with yourself. Drop all your defenses and ask what it is you want out of medicine— money? prestige? intangible rewards? If you answer this question truthfully then you can sort out your career."

Another student explained her decision-making process like this: "(1) Determine your priorities in life—family, prestige, time, money, academics, education, serving the populace, etc. (2) Decide what rotations you hated and why—then apply the explanation to other applicable specialties; for example, surgery, 'Because I can't stand to work all day with my hands.' That also rules out obstetrics, dermatology, and ophthalmology. (3) Of the rotations you liked, which best fits into your priorities? For instance, family is most important to me, and I like pediatrics best. So, I could work in a peds clinic or another nontraditional setting part-time while my children are growing up. I will make a smaller income, but money isn't my top priority."

You may be influenced by practitioners in that field: "A lot of it has to do with the professors you meet, somebody who impresses you, or a service where they let you do a lot." "You want to go where the dynamic personalities are. People are what make the specialty look good." "I'm going into surgery. I've always been close to my father, and he's a surgeon. When I was growing up, to me 'doctor' and 'surgeon' were synonymous."

Fourth-year students see different attractions in the specialties they've elected, ranging from personal convenience to intellectual and professional gratification. "Radiology won't distract me from my family and from what I like to do when I'm off the job." "I can go into pathology now without doing a medical or surgical internship. My children are still quite dependent and it upsets them when I have to stay out overnight or get called away." "Ophthal-mology is rated as a top specialty in terms of job satisfaction 5, 10, or 20 years after you get out into practice—both in enjoying your work and helping patients. And you have regular hours. You actually get the best of both worlds." "In ob/gyn, there's a whole lot of positive feedback. There aren't a bunch of chronically ill patients dying. It's a happier atmosphere."

Stereotypes of surgeons as self-assured and aggressive, impatient, and action-oriented are recognized by some students who describe their reasons for choosing a surgical specialty or subspecialty: "It's dramatic and it gets quick results." "If I were an internist rather than a surgeon, I'd sure hate to have to give up my patients for someone else to work on." One woman who had originally considered a surgical subspecialty said she finally decided against it because "There's a definite feeling among surgeons that it's a male stronghold. There are very few female surgeons. I think it's a pretty high-powered specialty, and you end up sacrificing a lot of things along the way." But "Women are finally breaking into surgery and there are women's support groups."

General practitioners and family practitioners tend to be seen as "nice types," hard workers, not necessarily at the top of their class academically, but very people oriented and concerned. One student took issue with this stereotype: "It's unfortunate that this idea is propagated, because general practice really requires the brightest people to go into it since there is such a wide body of medical knowledge to know." Family practice physicians have traditionally tended to be independent. They may not be as interested in earning top dollars as they are in knowing their patients and in occupying a position of respect in the community: "I come from a small town and I know the people. I know what general practice is like because of my parents' practice. I like working with people, and I like the social status of being known in the community. Money is not necessarily all that important." "I enjoy the variety. I don't like seeing one problem 15 or 20 times in a day. In family practice, you know that the next patient is going to be a little different." In recent years, primary care physicians have lost a measure of independence, but on the upside, family practice has also become more lucrative as the increasing need for primary care-givers has resulted in a financial shift in their favor.

People who choose internal medicine as a specialty share the same qualities as family practitioners. Although they remain concerned with the "total patient," they are perceived as being more scientifically oriented and concerned with a more detailed knowledge of disease processes. They are perceived as astute diagnosticians, intrigued by intellectual challenges. "I like sitting down and talking to somebody, thinking the problem out rather than just cutting on them and seeing what's wrong. I like the detective work." "I'm interested in doing research and teaching. I find internal medicine, even in a subspecialty like hematology, as a good opportunity to pursue a wide range of interests and to explore many different possibilities. I don't want to be confined to acute problems."

Pediatricians are almost universally characterized as "patient" and "good natured." It is widely agreed they must certainly enjoy children. Most people who choose this specialty talk in terms of the directness of their patients: "They don't hem and haw. You relieve their pain, they're happy. You make them hurt, they cry." "When you save a child's life, you can add over 60 years to the life span of this individual."

For some, psychiatry promises great rewards: "I've always been interested in this area, wanted to know why people tick." "I believe there's such a thing as mental health and, therefore, mental disease. And it's as serious as physical disease." "I've realized in working with patients these last few years that the emotional aspects of their problems and backgrounds are things I can't ignore. I get frustrated when I can't sit down and talk to a patient and let him ventilate a little bit." "You're like an explorer on a new frontier."

Aside from the initial decision to pursue a career in medicine, no other choice is likely to be as significant in the course of your professional life. If at the beginning stage in your training you feel overwhelmed by the prospect of making such an awesome decision, remember that the person who does the deciding will be someone very different from the person you are today. That person will have experienced a grueling, frustrating, and fascinating process that not only trains the mind and hands but also subtly probes and molds the character. That person will be not quite, but almost, a doctor!

Residency Interviews

Between September and December of your senior year you will don your most professional-looking garb and travel the country to be interviewed by directors of residency programs. You will want to secure a residency that will provide maximum exposure and training in your chosen field and will give you an opportunity to work with recognized specialists in that area. Obviously, certain institutions are preferable to others in each specialty area.

Choosing a residency involves more than just selecting the best place to receive additional training. For many graduating MDs, the years of residency offer an opportunity to "try out" the realities of practice in a new location: "Doing residency in a different part of the country will expose you to different philosophies of practice of medicine." Many students are eager to start fresh in new surroundings: "I can't imagine why anyone would want to stay here. I'm not used to staying in the same place for more than four years."

Prior to your interviews, the medical school dean will draft a letter of recommendation and mail it to the residency program directors you indicate. You will probably agonize about the contents of your letters and how well they will represent you to your prospective employers. Keep in mind, however, that no matter how important the paperwork, hospital directors generally consider the interview as the most important factor in evaluating potential residents.[5] This is what they look for, ranked from most to least important: (a) your personality, including maturity and stability; (b) expressed interest in their training program; (c) long-term career goals (e.g., research versus practice); (d) appearance; and (e) prediction of ability to solve clinical problems.

Program directors are biased against those who (a) desire only one year in the program—"Hospitals don't want an intern who is unsure, somebody who is just trying to get by for a year"; (b) ask about a reduced-schedule program; and (c) apply for specialties that differ from those they completed as electives. Be prepared to name your chosen specialty when you interview for residency appointments.

Being a team player is now critical. Keep this in mind as you prepare for your interview. If you are in a group interview and you try to stand out brilliantly "in fine competitive style, you may stand out primarily as being obnoxious. In residency, working well as part of a team is usually more valued than defeating, humiliating, or outshining your teammates."[6]

Keep in mind that the interview doesn't always go smoothly. "The interview lasts no more than 10 minutes, for which I flew 1500 miles."[7] When the AMSA Bioethics Task Force conducted a study of 225 fourth-year students attending the national convention concerning their interview experiences, 56% had been asked inappropriate questions that made them feel uncomfortable or discriminated against during their residency interview and 33% during their medical school interview. Women constituted nearly three fourths (72%) of those who had adverse interview experiences. Inappropriate questions often related to the applicants' gender, for example, women's traditional nurturing roles or plans for being both a mother and a doctor. The most blatant transgressions, however, came from the interviewer's behavior. One woman recalled, "The entire interview was spent with [the interviewer] staring at my breasts."

Questions regarding family planning accounted for 42% of the improprieties reported. Some of the questions were, "What kind of birth control are you planning to use during residency?" "When are you going to start having babies?" "Do you plan to have children during your medical training?" Perhaps most invasive of all, "If you got pregnant during medical school, what would you do?"[8] A woman who had finished her residency concluded this last question is appropriate, however: "Now that I've had to compensate for a colleague on maternity leave," she concluded, "I think it's legitimate to ask, 'Are you planning to take time off for pregnancy during the training period?' I don't think someone should lose a job over it, but everybody has to plan around the pregnancy."

Dr. Kenneth Iserson, a professor of surgery at the University of Arizona College of Medicine and author of *Getting Into a Residency: A Guide for Medical Students,* suggests these strategies for fielding off-limit questions: (a) Refuse to answer, perhaps stating that it is against the law to ask such questions or that it is none of the interviewer's business. Such a response is correct and legitimate, but will likely ensure that you don't get a residency position at that site. (b) Finesse the question by asking whether it is pertinent to obtaining a residency position. This gives the person, who probably has not been well trained to do this type of interviewing, a chance to back off and save face. Be very pleasant as you parry such questions. If you handle them deftly, correctly, you will still be a viable candidate for the program. Or (c) answer the question. This is what most applicants do in the medical field and other employment situations. This option may be distasteful, but it will not usually jeopardize your chances. Keep in mind that the interviewer may not even realize that he or she is violating both state and civil statutes.[9]

There are other problems. Students whose names indicate minority status may experience discrimination. For example, Adla Abdennabi, a fourth-year medical student at the University of Illinois College of Medicine sent 30 postcards to different internal medicine residency programs throughout the country. Two programs—both affiliated with a major institution in a large urban area in California—sent responses that shocked him. They refused to send him application materials simply because his name sounded foreign. One replied, "If you are not a native of the United States, we ask for proof that you are a legal resident of this country":

As a medical student, I have always heard rumors that applications from students with last names of some ethnic backgrounds are simply "circular filed." But the Attendings I have spoken to about this issue have reassured me that no such thing goes on. They all claim that they, at least, do not operate with such preconceived notions. But getting these letters has shown me that yes, when some programs I apply to receive my application, reading my name will be all that they will do before placing my application in the recycling bin.[10]

When you evaluate a residency program, try to talk with at least two other interns or residents currently enrolled in the program.[11] Find out how many interns are assigned to a clinical team. At some hospitals, teams consist of one intern and one resident and at other hospitals two interns and one resident. The latter is much better; it gives the residents twice as much help and the interns can help each other, share ideas, and commiserate about their experiences.

Is the program well organized with clearly stated objectives? You need to know what is expected of you and what you will be doing each month. Will you meet the guidelines of your specialty's governing board?

Does the residency program have a well-publicized evaluation system and grievance policy? A formal feedback process facilitates communication and lets you know how you are doing. It also helps keep up your morale when the workload seems overwhelming and you are discouraged that you are not making a difference. It is also important to know how you can provide supervisors with feedback about things that bother you. How do you appeal decisions that seem unfair? Avoid programs that orient new interns in a few minutes and then never discuss such topics again.

Is the hospital's allied health staff helpful? How willing are the nurses and other hospital personnel to help interns learn the ropes and assist you in your duties? If they are not supportive, it will mean increased interpersonal stress and more work for you. Do the physicians treat nurses and other allied health professionals condescendingly? If they do, the latter will likely be resentful and unwilling to help you.

Are days off scheduled and, if so, how many days per month or week? All residency programs purport to give house officers a minimum number of days off each month, but many do not actually schedule them in subtle pressure on interns and residents to work on their off days. You need an absolute minimum of at least four days a month of schedule-free time to count on if you are to avoid burnout and recuperate from the daily workload.

The Match

In March of your senior year, you will be assigned a residency through a computerized system known as the National Resident Matching Program (NRMP), which is administered by the Association of American Medical Colleges (AAMC) and governed by five sponsoring organizations. Student preferences are matched with potential training programs—ranked from the most to least preferred—with similar rankings of applicants by residency program directors. In 1995 and 1996, more than half of the U.S. seniors matched with a primary care program.[12] Each year, some students do not match. These students are notified by the medical school dean one or two days before the announcement so they can "scramble" (i.e., contact programs that did not fill and arrange an immediate match). Fortunately, some students make a better match this way than they originally applied for. Whatever the outcome, keep in mind that matching is *not* a definitive measure of your worth, accomplishments, or personality. It is just a computerized effort to achieve pairing of students and residency programs that sometimes doesn't work optimally.

Match Day is exciting! Envelopes are opened at the same time all across the country (noon on the East Coast and 9 a.m. on the West Coast). Some students tear open their envelope with family members and close friends at their side to find out where they will be for the next three to five years. Others go to a secluded place and open them in private. Excitement and congratulations fill the air as photographers circulate taking pictures, especially of those who have families present:

> After the Match Day, things feel different. The transition, which has been, for the past four years, almost impossible to imagine, has suddenly become real. We're all going to be doctors. When you have the name of the hospital, you can picture yourself working there. Not as a medical student, as a doctor.[13]

Insights: Coping With Criticism
Bernard Virshup, MD

Criticism is the medical school's primary way to help students learn, and they learn that nothing is ever done good enough. Few realize the depth of the average medical student's shame and humiliation when criticized in front of his or her peers or after failing at some task. It would not be so bad, except that the student's own inner critic agrees with everything negative that is said. The usual way in which the student copes with this is to establish a shell that as the years go by gets stronger and more brittle.

I deal with this in my workshops by giving students colored pastels and asking them to draw two fantasy animals on one sheet of paper. I say, "This is not an art class; it doesn't matter how well you draw. When you have your two animals, write three descriptive adjectives for each animal (a total of six adjectives). Then write a short story about the animals, starting with "Once upon a time."

Giving coloring material to students immediately regresses them to their childhood and they begin the exercise with every evidence of enjoyment. They look at each other's drawings and laugh. (How often do you hear medical students laugh?) Then, they write their three adjectives and their story and the room becomes very quiet. I ask if anyone has any ideas as to what this all means. Usually, someone ventures that it is in some way an expression of who they are. Right. I explain that when people draw two animals they almost always draw two different sides of themselves. For example, some will have drawn a heavy land animal and a bird—one side of themselves that is plodding and one side that wants to soar. And the adjectives they have written are, in some metaphorical sense, adjectives that describe two different parts of themselves.

Whoa! This gets their attention. They look at their drawings in a new light. I go on to explain that we all have an inherent sense of embarrassment at revealing ourselves to others. By revealing themselves to the other students, they now have a chance to face this sense of shame and embarrassment. It is a remarkably freeing experience to find that who we are is not so terrible to others and that everyone, although different, is basically similar. Then, I ask, who is willing to take the chance by showing us what he or she drew?

There is always one brave soul willing to show his or her picture and tell the adjectives and story. There is also inevitably appreciation, even applause, which encourages someone else, and then another, until finally everyone ends up sharing. Occasionally, I ask, "Does this have significance for you?" Sometimes, they say, "Oh, yes!" And sometimes, "I don't think so." But then, I say, "This is all very metaphorical; perhaps you can put it up on your refrigerator and look at if for a few days, and see if it doesn't have some meaning for you."

I explain further that there are many sides to us, not just one coherent self. Typically, we look at one side of us as bad, shameful, wrong; but there is always another side that is pretty good. When we feel ashamed of ourselves, what we need to do is to remember that there is another side of us that feels pretty good about ourselves. It's important to remember this. But it's hard to do and takes practice.

I go around the room and give them this needed practice. I simply ask them to repeat in some form whatever I say about them, to accept the part of them that agrees that this makes them feel bad, and then to find and express the other part that feels good about themselves.

For example, I usually start with the student next to me and say, "Your shoes are certainly scruffy looking!" If this totally confuses the student, I prompt, "Yes, there is a part of me that is ashamed of how they look, but there is another part of me that thinks I'm still a good person." I get the student to say it. He or she usually feels embarrassed, until I say to the next person, "I don't think that you should wear jeans to a medical school class." Again, there is difficulty responding, and I help by saying, "There is a part of me that agrees with you, but there is a bigger part of me that thinks it is perfectly O.K."

They get it. I go on to say something more meaningful to each student: "They really made a mistake when they let you into medical school." I patiently help the student find the answer, "Yes, there is a part of me that thinks that, but I know I'm going to be a good doctor." I say, "Women don't belong in medical school; it's a man's world here." That generally gets an angry response, and I use this to talk about anger and bigotry.

The important thing for the students to understand is that other people have thoughts that may or may not be valid but that they have a right to believe and express. Students need to be able to hear them and respond, "Well, I know that when you went into medicine there weren't many women, but we're really doing a great job!" I push them further by suggesting to the next student, "I don't think your last work-up was good enough; you'll never be a good doctor." By then, they usually can get to, "I know it wasn't as good as you or I would like, and you don't think I'll be a good doctor; that hurts, but basically what is important is that I'm enjoying what I'm doing, and I think I'll be a very good doctor." By now, the room is really getting into this.

Finally, I talk about "dexifying"—defending, explaining, and justifying—trying to convince the other person that I'm O.K. Don't do it, I urge; it doesn't work. Just let the other person be with his or her ideas, even when they hurt, and be comfortable with being who you are.

This process, called assertiveness training, is something that will help you live with yourself and with others. It is something that needs continual reinforcement throughout an entire lifetime.

Notes

1. Daugherty, Steven R., and DeWitt C. Baldwin, Jr. 1996, January. "Sleep Deprivation in Senior Medical Students and First-Year Residents." *Academic Medicine,* 71(1):S93-S95.

2. Oryshkevich, Bohdan. 1992. "Are We Mortgaging the Medical Profession?" (Letter to the editor). *New England Journal of Medicine,* 326(4):274-275.

3. Cohn, Arlan, and Aka Oscar London. 1992, February 24-28. "How to Be the World's Best Doctor." Presented at UCSD School of Medicine conference, Physician Heal Thyself, San Diego, CA.

4. Iserson, Kenneth V. 1996. *Getting Into A Residency: A Guide for Medical Students.* Tucson, AZ: Galen.

5. Zerega, W. Dennis, and Bruce Deighton. 1991. *Selecting the Right Residency for You: A Decision Making Guide* (2nd ed.). Author.

6. Krogh, Christopher. 1986, October. "Residency Interviews: A Closer Look." *The New Physician,* pp, 33-45, p. 34.

7. Ciesielski-Carlucci, Chris, Gene Hern, and Thomasine K. Kushner. 1995, November. "A Right Gone Wrong." *The New Physician,* pp. 23-26, p. 23.

8. *Ibid.*

9. Iserson, *op. cit.*

10. Abdennabi, Adla. 1995, October. "What's in a Name?" (Letter to the editor). *The New Physician,* p. 3.

11. Knudsen, Christie. 1996, November. "Choice Questions." *The New Physician,* pp. 21-22.

12. Tschida, Molly. 1996, May-June. "Match of the Day." *The New Physician,* p. 7.

13. Klass, Perri. 1986, January. "Now We Are All Going to Be Doctors." *Discover,* pp. 14, 16; p. 14.

CHAPTER 9

Graduation
What Happens Next?

Very little of my work as a physician was glamorous in the TV drama sense, but much of it was intense. Daily I was tossed from sore throat to heart attack, from psychosomatic illness to life-threatening emergency, from birth to death. Each patient required my full emotional involvement, my full energy. Even an apparently minor illness could bring an unexpected challenge, for serious illness or injury can lurk behind any seemingly innocuous symptom. I had to be constantly on guard.[1]

—Family physician

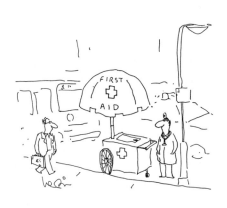

Receiving a medical degree, a momentous milestone, marks the beginning of yet another turn at the bottom of the hierarchical ladder. For most graduates, it also means moving, often to a different part of the country, and another experience of learning the ropes. Your new status means longer hours, hard work, greater pressure, and increased responsibility for patient care. This time fewer people will be supervising you.

Postgraduate work is the ultimate in hands-on apprenticeship. You will have the highest quality of relevant experience and the opportunity to work with outstanding role models. By now, you will have some fairly definite ideas about the kind of physician you want to become in terms of specialty and in the broader sense of being a "good doctor." You will have developed criteria to satisfy that definition, and you may still fall short of your own standards.

Drawing by Levin; © 1988 The New Yorker Magazine, Inc.

The Residency Years

Residency training varies depending on specialty. During your first year, postgraduate year 1 (PGY-1), you will complete an internship in internal medicine, surgery, pediatrics, or another field. Then, during PGY-2, PGY-3, and so on, you will become more deeply involved in your specialty training. Family medicine, the shortest, requires four years, including internship; some surgical residencies may take seven. Additional subspecialty fellowships can extend your training an additional one to four years beyond residency.

If you are a U.S. student who attended medical school outside of the United States, you must pass qualifying exams and complete an extra year of clinical training, called a "fifth pathway year," to qualify for a residency. After you have invested enormous personal resources in foreign training, sometimes requiring a new language, adapting to different customs, and perhaps experiencing prejudice and discrimination, you may be one of the fortunate ones accepted for this fifth year of clinical training. The so-called doctor glut has focused negative attention on foreign medical schools and reduced the number of opportunities to practice in the United States.

Your residency will be your most significant rite of passage. Now, you are an MD (a medical school graduate), and you will become an "RD" (real doctor). In medical school, you learned the basic vocabulary and syntax necessary to perform as an orthodox physician, and now the weight of personal responsibility will be yours and you will feel it keenly. The level of your clinical skills and any personal deficits will become strikingly apparent to you.

You will work as a member of a floor team. An attending physician serves as mentor and teacher. The team includes a senior resident (someone in the last year of training), several junior residents (those in their second or third year, depending on the program's length), interns, and a number of medical students and nurses. Maintaining good rapport with each is important.

Although you became acquainted with this collaboration during your clinical clerkships, as a new physician you will relate to other team members differently. You give orders to nurses now, so be careful not to alienate them with a know-it-all attitude. Treat them with utmost courtesy and respect, as collaborators, not underlings. They generally have a lot more experience. Listen to them. You need them on your side. They can help you or make life miserable for you. The following behaviors really irritate nurses: (a) "borrowing" things (e.g., a nurse's stethoscope) and not returning them promptly, (b) expecting nurses to clean up after you, (c) interfering with nurses' work by lounging at their station or tying up their telephone, and (d) asking nurses to drop whatever they are doing to do scut work for you (e.g., calling the lab for test results).[2] Don't assume that your time is more valuable or your work any more important than theirs.

The Internship (PGY-1)

The dictionary defines an intern as an inmate, one confined or detained within the limits of a specific place. Historically, interns and residents resided in the hospital. They received no salary, just board and room. In return, they were granted, as apprentices to the attending physicians, the privilege of caring for patients. Much has changed. House staff now receive salaries and no longer reside exclusively in the hospital (there are still some places where the traditional pattern exists, such as the trauma team rotation at a San Francisco hospital where the chief resident resides at the hospital for a month's time). Even though residents have their own private quarters, the residency is highly confining. Most of your time will be spent in the hospital, especially when you are on call. Sleep will be a luxury.

The typical hospital intern works every weekday and spends every third night on duty. You may work a hectic 36-hour shift at least twice a week. On a bad night, you may not sleep, and your income, when divided by the hours worked, approximates the minimum wage.

Work schedules of 90 to 120 hours a week may leave you feeling isolated and physically and emotionally exhausted. Because there is little time to digest new information or talk with others who are experiencing the same challenges, interns often weather the experience alone, without knowing how they are doing or how others are doing.

Perri Klass described her first night on call as "terror, exhilaration, and exhaustion." Her first patient was a newborn who weighed less than three pounds, requiring her to

> bumble around the intensive care unit, which is a complex place set up to make it possible for a large group of highly trained adults to take care of a group of very sick, very small babies. And of course I don't know where anything is. I can't find the pencil sharpener, I can't find the cardiac resuscitation medications. I can't even fill out the x-ray form correctly, which is no joke when you want them to come take an emergency x-ray of a desperately sick baby and they reject your form. I try to get my work done, pausing every few minutes to get a nurse, or the ward secretary, or

anyone at all, to show me where to find some crucial items. "Trust the nurses. They know what they're doing, they're the only ones who do," advised a friend who has already completed several years of residency. And it's true.[3]

Whether you are outside the hospital corridors for a change of scenery or some fresh air or immersed in patient care or paperwork, the ever-present beeper will summon you back. Although these electronic gadgets enhance communication, they add stress to a frenzied life. A senior resident commented:

> I just hate being in the middle of working up a patient in the E.R. and just about ready to listen to the heart or whatever and the beeper goes off and I have to trot off to the nearest phone to find out what's wanted. Since there isn't a phone nearby, I have to traipse down the hall to the closest telephone, and just as you are thinking you might be able to figure out the poor guy in the E.R., there's someone in the ICU who also needs your immediate attention. And then, as you are walking back down the hall to the E.R., the beeper goes off again! It's very stressful to hear. Three to four different interns may need a urology consult now, and you need to respond. It's hard to remain unruffled inwardly, as well as outwardly, when constantly interrupted.[4]

Good time management is important when the beeper incessantly sounds off. Robert Lowes suggests assigning tasks to four categories: (a) urgent and important, (b) urgent but not important, (c) not urgent but important, and (d) not urgent and not important. By cutting back on the latter tasks (e.g., talking to drug representatives), you will have more time for important but nonurgent tasks (e.g., studying for a new rotation).[5]

In an article titled "Survival Training," Lowes cautions, "Make no mistake about it," the first year of residency training is "a baptism by fire. . . . It's okay to burst into tears after your third day as an intern and wonder why you ever wanted to be a doctor."[6] He advises you to gather some commonsense advice about internship before you begin but warns that it will be impossible to be in control of your circumstances and to be tearless and fearless:

> The best way to get ready is by recognizing with your human limitations. Such realism will go a long way as you sit at your patient's bedside, hear

advice from nurses, play quiz-show with attending physicians, and try to maintain your own health despite grueling call schedules. Treat everyone with dignity and be willing to say "I don't know."[7]

Prerounding on patients in the early morning before official rounds with attendings is important and includes finding out lab results and locating X rays. "Use index cards or a hand-held computer to record or update patient data," advises a residency director. "But whatever you do, write every thing down. Don't rely on memory. You'll be too tired, and it will fail you."[8]

When attending physicians yell at you, don't take it personally. "If it's vicious, just point out that the comments are inappropriate and undeserved. But don't attack or humiliate the attending physician in front of your team. If the problem is serious, go through channels, such as the chief resident." Another resident adds, "The best thing to do is take them aside and ask, 'I'm working hard. What brought this on?'"[9]

Residency Burnout

Most of the trials and tribulations of the internship year continue into subsequent years of training. New stressors and new sources of satisfaction may emerge. For one thing, residents (PGY-2 and beyond) are more accountable than interns for the ultimate progress of patients—the "buck" stops with them. Residents also do more teaching than interns; they supervise both medical students and interns. For some residents, teaching is challenging and exciting. For others, it is an additional responsibility and burden.

Residency training reinforces typical physician attributes—conscientiousness, responsibility, and willingness to work long hours—that sometimes cause physical and emotional exhaustion or even psychiatric disorders. House officers' attempts to ameliorate depression, common among them, can lead to dependence on alcohol or other drugs. The importance of maintaining supportive relationships as a buffer against these unpleasant possibilities cannot be overemphasized. Rather than stuffing your feelings, open up with somebody who you can trust—a spouse, parent, sibling, or intimate friend. "In my mind there's nothing that helps me maintain my personal equilibrium better than some time at home with wife, family and friends."[10] Even when you are on call, take time to phone someone who cares about you as a person—not just as a doctor—someone who will let you blow off steam about your circumstances, your frustrations.

A resident's schedule may consist of shifts of 36 hours on duty and 8 off, followed by 12 hours on and 12 off, then starting again with a 36-hour shift. Resident advocacy groups for years have struggled to reform these working conditions. They criticize the traditional system for failing to address the debilitating effects of sleep deprivation. Research shows that exhausted doctors make more mistakes, lose compassion for patients, and have more conflicts with staff.[11] Moreover, they argue, the grueling pace of residency training wrecks havoc with a physician's personal life. Andy Nowalk asks how "we can be effective healers and ministers to others when we completely neglect our own lives."[12] Some residents are philosophical: "I look upon residency training as a self-limited disease. It will go away with time. Eventually you'll get back to your pre-morbid self. Your sense of humanism will return to you."[13]

Fortunately, not everyone experiences a miserable time in residency. Some say of their residency, even though "interspersed with sleepless nights, intellectual demands, and emotional challenges, the ultimate effect was surprisingly and unambiguously beneficent."[14] Malcontents aren't the only ones who publish memoirs about their residencies. William Noonan's experience was "an emotionally rewarding as well as intellectually stimulating experience for me and my fellow house officers."[15] At the small hospital—13 interns and 16 upper-level residents—where he trained, house officers were treated with courtesy and respect by faculty, medical attendings, nurses, and staff. This, he says, was in sharp contrast to the incivility that he experienced as a medical student at a large university hospital, "where internecine warfare was sometimes waged between and within the levels of the hospital hierarchy."[16]

In Noonan's residency, trainees were encouraged to pay attention to their emotions as a way to provide better patient care. At a weekly house staff support meeting, led by a psychiatrist-facilitator, residents shared frustrations, discussed anxieties about their roles, and proposed solutions to their common problems. They could talk about the tragedy of death; the sometimes-irrational behavior of patients; and the competing demands of family, friends, patients, colleagues, and teachers.[17] Several times a year, the noon teaching conference was devoted to sharing "critical incidents." Faculty and house staff described events in their medical and postgraduate educations that left indelible and sometimes painful memories. These conferences encouraged trainees to recognize the pain that is an inherent part of practicing medicine and reassured them that they were not alone in facing uncomfortable issues.[18]

The faculty also used spontaneous opportunities to emphasize the importance of a physician's affective responses to tragedy and death. When a young patient of Noonan's died unexpectedly, an attending physician stopped by to talk about the experience:

> He asked if this was the first patient I had had die and how I felt about it. I shrugged bravely, donned my mantle of professional detachment, and lied, saying I was handling it well. Diplomatically overlooking my transparent denial, he started to talk about the importance of acknowledging the sense of loss we can feel as physicians when a patient dies. He encouraged me not to ignore the discomfort, but instead to confront it and learn to live with it. Any other course, he said, would only leave emotional scars that would accumulate over the years and dull my enjoyment of the profession.[19]

The ideal residency, one sensitive to the needs of residents as well as their patients, should be the right of *every* trainee, not the exception. In 1957, the Committee of Interns and Residents formed the oldest and largest house staff union in the United States. Housed in New York (386 Park Avenue South, Room 1502, New York, NY 10016; 212/725-5500), the union organizes collective bargaining to guarantee house staff rights, reduce work hours, protect residency health and safety, establish maternity leave rights, advocate high-quality patient care, improve salaries and benefits, defend staffing levels, and speak out on health care reform.

New York, which trains about 15% of the nation's doctors, was the first state to legislate changes in residency education. Effective July 1, 1989, the New York Department of Health amended section 405 of the state hospital code with a set of regulations that slashed the number of hours that residents in some specialties could be allowed to work and increased their supervision while on duty. It assured residents of an 80-hour work week, a continuous 24-hour period off each week, a minimum of 8 hours off between shifts, and around-the-clock supervision by fully trained physicians. These changes improved the quality of life for medical residents and the quality of health care provided by the state's teaching hospitals.[20] More than 60% of residents and attendings say that patients receive better care as a result of increased supervision.

In 1990, the California Association of Interns and Residents (CAIR, Tel. 310/632-0111), an organization that bargains in behalf of California resident physicians and represents about a quarter of them, signed an affiliation agreement with the Service Employees International Union (SEIU). This affiliation with SEIU is the first time nationally that physicians-in-training have joined forces with an AFL-CIO member union.[21]

Pregnancy

All residents experience difficulties in maintaining viable personal lives. But a married women resident can have an additional layer of stressors. She may feel pressure to take on "the second shift," of homemaking and child care. Many hire nannies. "Everybody needs a wife," one remarked, "especially a married female resident."

In 1996, women made up 42% of medical school entrants.[22] So, by the turn of the century, 42% of residents will be female. A nationwide survey of women in ob/gyn, psychiatry, and surgery residencies found that 31% had a child during their residency.[23] Teaching hospitals are increasingly responding to the needs of these women. In 1994, Ingrid Philibert and Janet Bickel sent a 20-item questionnaire to 405 Council of Teaching Hospitals (COTH) of the AAMC for detailed and up-to-date information about maternity and other parental-leave policies.[24] With a 45% response rate, over three fourths indicate having written policies that specify maternity or parental leave for house staff, a significant increase since 1989, when only around one half of the hospitals who reported had written policies of this type. Of the 42 hospitals who reported no written policy (23%), 27 indicated that house staff requesting maternity or parental leave used other categories of leave to serve as parental leave. The average maximum days of maternity leave allowed was 63.7 days, with a range of 21 to 180 days.

What happens when a female resident is pregnant? Having a baby at this busy time often evokes resentment from program directors and fellow residents. So, realizing that her colleagues (other harried house staff) must take on the additional burden of her undone work, she may not take the time for herself that she would advise her own patients. Also, medical knowledge may stimulate anxiety. A physician is more acutely aware than others of what can go wrong and of the various risks, such as infection, difficult deliveries, and the possibility of a damaged or stillborn baby.[25]

It is to be hoped that the trend of written parental leave policies will continue until all hospitals have well-formulated maternity, paternity, and adoption leave. This will reduce stress and clarify expectations for those who need such leave and their fellow residents.

Fellowship Training

After your residency training, you may opt to pursue additional specialized training as a fellow in subspecialties such as thoracic surgery, child psychiatry, endocrinological gynecology, or ultrasound radiology. Internal medicine, for example, offers a variety of subspecialty training opportunities, just a few of which are gastroenterology, hematology, cardiology, and rheumatology. Fellowships last one to four years and provide in-depth clinical experience in a specialized field of medicine.

Fellows earn roughly the same amount as residents, but they often supplement their income by moonlighting, that is, working at a second job after hours or on days off. Generally, they are not free to set up a private practice. Fellows remain under the supervision of the department chairperson and are subject to the policies that regulate other house officers.

What motivates residents to add additional years to an already lengthy training period? You may feel the need for more in-depth training or want to delineate a narrower area of clinical expertise. Or you may not feel ready for independent private practice, want to develop an academic track, or enhance your future income or prestige. It's a sure way to keep up with increased technological developments and to successfully compete for patients.

The fellow's lifestyle is typically more relaxed than that of an intern or resident. Rather than working 60 to 100 hours a week, a fellow's workweek is closer to 40 to 70 hours. Although clinical work is expected, especially in tertiary care centers, or when the department chairperson lacks confidence in the residents, for the most part the workload is lighter. For instance, fellows no longer have the responsibility of admitting new patients.

This time may be opportune for starting a family if you haven't already or to catch up on other neglected matters.

Medical Practice

After a prolonged training period requiring four years of undergraduate work, four years of medical school, and three to seven years of residency training, you will finally leave the confines of the teaching hospital to venture forth into the world at large. This shift from dependence to independence, although eagerly anticipated, may not be easy. You will be repaying financial, marital, and emotional debts and starting something new. Unfortunately, little is said or done in medical school or postgraduate training to prepare you for this relatively uncharted course.

If you picture yourself in a nice little office with a steady flow of patients and just your name on the door, you may be disillusioned. "In the old days," a surgery resident notes,

> the doctor decided why, when and how to treat patients. Nobody asked questions or challenged medical decisions. The interaction between doctor and patient was almost holy. A treatment plan was determined in the privacy of the doctor's office, and nobody could interfere with its execution. Those days are over.[26]

Paperwork and other pressures have become so overwhelming that solo practitioners are forced to join a larger organization or build their own by hiring clerks and teaming up with other doctors to form groups large enough to contract with health insurers. One physician laughed, "It's easier to get butterflies to fly in formation than to organize physicians."[27] For a steady paycheck, a manageable call schedule, and freedom from administrative tasks and paperwork required by insurance companies, joining an HMO may be your choice. Currently, physicians working in HMOs outnumber solo practitioners and this trend is accelerating.[28]

Health insurance companies now demand a say in virtually every physician procedure. Precertification, instigated by insurance companies individually during the mid-1980s, coincided with the arrival of Medicare's diagnostic-related groups (DRGs), which capped reimbursements.

Managed care in its various forms has changed the practice of medicine. According to Dr. Doug Campos-Outcalt, director of the family practice residency program at Maricopa Medical Center in Phoenix, managed care is "not just the practice of medicine under new restraints . . . it's a new way of doing things."[29]

With the growth of managed care, doctors' authority and pay have dwindled. For example, one cardiologist who had it all—money, prestige, and a thriving medical practice—suffered when his contract with a giant health insurer was pulled and his patients switched to another cardiology group willing to work more cheaply. He lost 3,000 patients and half of his income and faced foreclosure on his home. His $70,000 Mercedes—the doctor's symbol of success—was sold, and he sought a bankruptcy lawyer. "This is destroying me," he said. "I feel like I wasted my time in school and I'm not of any value anymore."[30]

Managed care as defined by the Princeton economist Uwe Reinhardt is the "external proctoring and micro-managing of the ongoing doctor-patient relationship on the basis of predetermined practice guidelines"; "capitation" shifts "some or all of the financial risk of a patient's illness onto the shoulders of physicians who make the treatment decisions."[31]

For generations, the fundamental relationship in medicine was between doctor and patient. Now, it includes three parties: the doctor, the patient, and the bureaucrats who play a powerful role in how medicine is financed and practiced. About 100 million Americans are in some type of managed care and 76% of doctors contract with managed care companies. A surgery resident notes,

> The advent of managed care has made every treatment decision subject to negotiation. There is pre-approval for hospital admissions and surgical interventions. There are limits on length of stay in the hospital. There are constraints on which medicines may be prescribed. There are restrictions on when and why to obtain specialist consultation. . . . A colleague of mine is a neurosurgeon. He once did a complicated surgery to remove a brain tumor. The patient's managed-care plan approved one day in the intensive-care unit following the surgery. That day came and went. The patient still had uneven breathing. Her blood pressure and heart rate continued to fluctuate dangerously, as is often the case after the brain is manipulated in surgery. The doctor decided she needed another day in the ICU: She still needed minute-by-minute monitoring and physiologic fine-tuning.
>
> The doctor phoned her HMO to obtain approval for the extra day of ICU care. The HMO's utilization-review nurse consulted a guide book that outlined the HMO's policies for allowable treatments. It stated only one day was allowed in the ICU. So she denied the extra day. The doctor felt that it would be medically unacceptable to transfer the patient out of the ICU. He kept her there. The next day he was called by another utilization-review nurse from the HMO. She explained that since the second day of ICU care had not been approved, its cost would be deducted from his surgeon's fee. "You'd better transfer the patient out today," she warned. Then she made a joke: "If these ICU costs keep adding up, the deductions will surpass your fee. Not only won't you get paid for caring for the patient, you could wind up owing us money."[32]

You may receive some managed care training. More and more medical schools are teaching about these health care systems.[33] In 1997, the Pew Charitable Trusts set up a multimillion-dollar initiative to develop partnerships between academic health centers and managed care organizations.[34] Young physicians find themselves in a heavily managed care environment. "They need to know their options," notes Barbara Barzansky, assistant director of AMA's division of undergraduate education. "If they've never had any training in managed care, how can they decide if this is where they want to work?"[35]

In 1996, the University of California appointed a commission of medical scholars to address the conflict "between the way doctors are taught to practice and the way they are forced to practice due to sweeping changes in managed care."[36] Called the Commission on the Future of Medical Education, the 28-person commission recommended that more emphasis must be placed on teaching business skills and that students be trained in other settings as well as in hospitals. "We are seeing the death of a cottage industry and the birth of the industrialization of medicine," said one commissioner. "For the first time, we're in a world where demand will drive employment. . . . We're not far away from ophthalmologists driving taxicabs. The idea of sending out graduates to set up shop is no longer possible."[37]

A new approach to medical education is a matter of survival, a neurosurgeon noted: "We have to deal with the realities here. There are those who think we are abrogating our mission if we turn into a trade school. But it's not an either/or decision. We've been producing what we want to produce, not what we need."[38]

Traditional medical training has been based on diagnosing and treating disease. But future doctors will need business and computer skills. "We grew up in an era of 'You name your price, and they will pay it,'" a commissioner noted. "But that is gone forever."[39] Understanding the human body and disease processes may become less important than it once was as physicians increasingly seek treatment plans from computer databases.

According to the commission's report, doctors of the future will "direct teams that include nurses, nurse practitioners, midwives, physician's assistants, osteopaths, nutritionists, and behavioral specialists such as social workers." "Eighty percent of what doctors do can be done by nurses and physician's assistants," said one physician commissioner. According to the commission, medical schools must deal with such challenging issues as (a) reducing the number of physicians, particularly specialists, because HMOs assign more patient care to nurses, physicians' assistants, and other personnel;

(b) teaching medical students business and computer skills they will need; and (c) meeting increasing demand for alternative care methods including psychological, nutritional, and spiritual foundations of health. Alternative care methods, another commissioner noted, "were not even on the radar screen in the 70's in medical school. We have been demeaning preventive health for years," another added. "Medical students can't fall asleep in epidemiology and nutrition classes."[40]

What does the future hold for physicians? Eli Ginzberg of Columbia University sees these developing trends: (a) increased, but slower-paced enrollment in managed-care plans; (b) a significant decline in beds in acute care hospitals; (c) a rise in the number of uninsured; and (d) a rise in the nation's health care expenditures. He also predicts that (a) physicians' income will decline and some may be unemployed; (b) physicians treating patients with health insurance will be compelled to consider cost versus benefits of diagnostic and therapeutic procedures; (c) most physicians will be working to a greater extent as members of medical teams with support staff who will have expanded assignments; and (d) there will be more discontent in the health care sector of our society.[41] Nevertheless, as Reinhardt points out, although the "golden days of medicine are history . . . the perennial intellectual challenge of medicine remains and so does the capacity to do immense good"; there are, he notes, "awesome psychic rewards."[42] "While some older doctors may be demoralized," comments the same surgery resident cited earlier, "many young doctors like me go to work each day with enthusiasm. The excitement of the job's clinical challenges offsets the bureaucratic hurdles imposed by managed-care plans."[43]

Retirement

You probably laughed when you first noticed the heading for retirement, a topic too far into the future to even consider. But, like a farmer plowing, you'll save time and energy—cut a straighter furrow—if you have a long-term perspective.

Retired physicians looking back on their careers emphasize the importance of maintaining interests outside of medicine. The most successful retirees developed other interests. "My list of interests is so long it's astounding," one said. "There are so many enjoyable things to do that there just isn't enough time." "Looking back, I don't know how I've found time to practice medicine," another added. These physicians look with pity on those who devote themselves fully to their practice: "They are so preoccupied with medicine their interest in other things is zero. Doctors who devote themselves to their careers don't realize that when they die, society won't skip a beat. No one's going to miss them."

For those who live only for their careers, retirement can be painful. Those whose self-image relies solely on career attainment feel an inevitable loss of self-worth on retiring. "When I retired I was at a loss," one related, "My self-esteem took a real beating." Nobody came for advice, no one seemed to look up to him as special. "What am I worth now?" he wondered. "I went from being almost worshipped to just an ordinary guy."

Many retired physicians regret having neglected their families. "I was a father who left home at 5 a.m. and returned between 8 p.m and midnight, long after the children's bedtime. I wasn't that involved in their lives. I was a semi-stranger to them. I wish I had been there more and given them more support." These doctors regret missing out on significant moments in their children's development: "I knew very little about what my kids were doing. I rarely ate a meal with them."

Empty-shell marriages—those that survive but lack emotional vitality—can be poignant for retired physicians who gave their all to medicine. "I found that if you don't love your spouse when you retire, you're in a mess," one observed. "As long as you have love, each other, and get along, you're alright." Doctors who take time to cultivate healthy marital relationships through the years welcome the additional time afforded at retirement to spend together. And their relationship even improves. "She's one remarkable person," one doctor acknowledged. "I've been fortunate. I honestly look forward to the free time that we spend together." "My spouse is one fantastic person, really! I don't know how the hell I got that lucky."

Let me emphasize again, as I have throughout this book, that the simplest and most profound way to maintain your mental health at any stage—while actively involved in intense training; during a demanding, open-ended career; or in retirement—is to establish and cultivate viable relationships with family members. Lack of companionship is an interpersonal deficit that makes you vulnerable to stress. At work, you are judged primarily on the basis of your achievements. On good days, that can be very rewarding. On bad days, however, it can be devastating. Fortunately, mates and other family members place more emphasis on *who you are* than on *what you can do*. Emotionally supportive relationships, such as that provided within a caring family, can sustain you through difficult times.

Like careers, interpersonal relationships must be carefully nurtured. A prominent senior physician expressed it this way:

> Most doctors don't realize what is happening to their marriages until they get to their 40s and by that time they have lost contact with their families. Upon seeing that the road to glory is going to end and that they are achieving the thing they have striven for, their disappointment is bitter to find success is really cotton candy; there is no substance to it. The thing that is really important—their interpersonal relationships with family members—has gone down the drain.

Health and happiness can be lost through overwork, perfectionism, and excessive career zeal. Become a "compleat" physician, one who has balanced head (intellect), hands (clinical skills), and heart (emotional expressiveness).

The most successful physicians, those who enjoy their work and find fulfillment, maintain a healthy balance between work, family life, and other activities. These compleat physicians are in contrast to "impaired doctors" who, although technically competent, are neither balanced nor comfortable with the socioemotional aspects of their work and personal lives. Overwork and emotional isolation seem to be at the core of physician impairment. Excessive work results not only from outside demands but from internal needs such as competitiveness and excessive thoroughness. Pursuing excellence and constantly trying to impress a critical audience (primarily other physicians) can skew the doctor's lifestyle in the direction of excessive career involvements. Chronically overworked and preoccupied, physicians can become physically and emotionally exhausted, with anxiety, irritability, and depression as predictable manifestations. As they chronically suppress feelings of anxiety, doubt, and inadequacy, emotions that cry for expression, physicians easily become unbalanced. Depression, chemical dependence, and even suicide occur far too frequently.[44]

There is little in medical education or practice to develop emotional expressiveness. Usually, clinicians are expected to remain analytical and emotionally aloof in this historically male-dominated milieu. Such composure—machismo—may be highly valued but is personally and interpersonally emotionally dysfunctional. Patients want a doctor who is skilled and who shows concern and a genuine interest in their welfare.[45] How can a physician show warmth to patients when he or she chronically neglects self-care? "The longer I live," Oliver Wendell Holmes observes, the more I am satisfied of two things: first, that the truest lives are those that are cut rose-diamond fashion, with many faces answering to the many planed aspects of the world about them; secondly, that society is always trying in some way or other to grind us down to a single flat surface. It is hard work to resist this grinding down action.[46]

Compleat physicians balance their activities to avoid physical and emotional exhaustion:

There is a two-fold opposition to a well-balanced life: (1) One is simply our own failure to determine the values we want in life, and how much each effort should receive. (2) The second is the social pressure that favors one or more of these values to the exclusion of others.[47]

"What men attempt," Bernard Baruch observed, "they seem driven to overdo."[48] This potential for extremes and excess marks many human endeavors, but it reaches an art form among some physicians.

If you attend to your self-care, keeping a healthy balance between career and family, you will do better, not worse in your career activities. Picture the columns on a financial ledger. Success is not measured by high attainment in only one column, especially if it is achieved at the expense of the other columns; it must be measured horizontally—by assessing all the important elements. Compleat physicians consider all dimensions of their lives. They do not admire their colleagues who, although they obtain honorific professional status, have done so at the expense of their personal and familial well-being.

Take time to keep your family relationships viable. In Maslow's "hierarchy of human needs,"[49] the need for love and belonging immediately follows that for food and shelter. Of the various mechanisms that society has established to meet this need, marriage and family are the most universal and can be, with planning and effort, the most fulfilling.

Insights: Balancing Professional Excellence
With Personal and Social Well-Being
Bernard Virshup, MD

The good physician excels not only professionally. If, in the pursuit of professional excellence, you neglect activities that are emotionally enriching, you increase your proneness to emotional bankruptcy. The good physician in addition to being knowledgeable and skilled attends to his or her personal and social well-being. Personal well-being and professional excellence are not mutually exclusive; both are necessary, and at the same time!

Among the needs we must fill for a successful and satisfying medical career and life are the following: warm, intimate, supportive relationships; exercise, rest, good nutrition, and recreation; a solidly based good sense of self and of self-worth not entirely dependent on success, achievements, or the opinions of others; an ability to accept imperfection, failures, and mistakes in ourselves and others; an ability to relate comfortably with patients; an openness to our feelings—good and bad—and an ability to cope well with the latter. Sounds good? Certainly. Easy to achieve? Certainly not. In fact, many physicians never achieve these goals. Why? Medicine does not lend itself easily to the well-being of the physician. The medical mystique implies that good doctors are dedicated to their work to the exclusion of all other considerations and willing to work under conditions of stress and long hours that would fell mere mortals.

Medicine and life are necessarily stressful. Nevertheless, I do not believe that these stresses are inevitably detrimental. Stress lies less in the situation in which we find ourselves than in the way we perceive that situation, the meaning it has for us personally, and what we do about it. Many physicians make good decisions about the amount of work they will do and manage to live well-balanced, full lives and enjoy medicine. Many people who are stressed use the opportunity to improve their coping skills and to grow psychologically. In my medical education, physician well-being was often neglected or actively deprecated. One reason, it has been said, is that medicine is a jealous lover that begrudges us the time and energy to fill our own essential needs. Perhaps, it is time to change that relationship. It is time to start taking care of yourself and of the people who care for you. It is time to start enjoying your patients as *people*. It is time to start enjoying medicine. It is time to start enjoying your life.

Notes

1. Hilfiker, David. 1985. *Healing the Wounds.* New York: Pantheon, p. 25.

2. Lowes, Robert. 1996, March. "Survival Training." *The New Physician,* pp. 21-24, p. 22.

3. Klass, Perri. 1986, September. "First Night On-Call: Terror, Exhilaration, Exhaustion." *Discover,* pp. 18-19, p. 19.

    4. Coombs, Robert H., D. Scott May, and Gary W. Small, eds. 1986. *Inside Doctoring: Stages and Outcomes in the Professional Development of Physicians.* New York: Praeger, p. 82.

    5. Lowes, *op. cit.*

    6. *Ibid.,* p. 21.

    7. *Ibid.,* pp. 21-22.

    8. *Ibid.,* p. 23.

    9. *Ibid.,* p. 22.

    10. Nowalk, Andy. 1997, January-February. "Home Free." *The New Physician,* p. 44.

    11. Daugherty, Steven R., and Dewitt C. Baldwin, Jr. 1996, January supplement. "Sleep Deprivation in Senior Medical Students and First-Year Residents." *Academic Medicine,* 71(1):S93-S95.

    12. Nowalk, *op. cit.*

    13. Marion, Robert. 1991. *Learning to Play God: The Coming of Age of a Young Doctor.* Reading, MA: Addison-Wesley.

    14. Noonan, William D.M. 1995, Summer. "Must An Internship Be Miserable?" *The Pharos,* pp. 19-23, p. 19.

    15. *Ibid.*

    16. *Ibid.,* p. 20.

    17. *Ibid.*

    18. *Ibid.*

    19. *Ibid.,* p. 20.

    20. Chollar, Susan. 1991, July-August. "Resident Relief." *The New Physician,* pp. 18-23.

    21. Williams, Linda Darnell. 1990, November 5. "Interns Are RX for Better Care." *Los Angeles Times,* pp. D1, D8.

    22. Philibert, Ingrid, and Janet Bickel. 1995. "Maternity and Parental Leave Policies at COTH Hospitals: An Update." *Academic Medicine,* 70:1055-1058.

    23. Phelan, S. 1992. "Sources of Stress and Support for the Pregnant Resident." *Academic Medicine,* 67:408-410.

    24. Philibert and Bickel, *op. cit.*

    25. Trupin, Suzanne. 1986. "When the Obstetrician Gets Pregnant." In Robert H. Coombs, D. Scott May, and Gary W. Small, eds. *Inside Doctoring: Stages and Outcomes in the Professional Development of Physicians* (pp. 131-133). New York: Praeger.

    26. Krieger, Lloyd M. 1997, June 1. "The HMO (Attrition) Plan: It's Doctor vs. Bureaucracy." *Los Angeles Times,* p. M1.

    27. Tschida, Molly. 1996, December. "Managed Care 101." *The New Physician,* pp. 23-29, p. 29.

    28. Kletke, Phillip R., David W. Emmons, and Kurt D. Gillis. 1996. "Current Trends in Physicians' Practice Arrangements." *Journal of the American Medical Association,* 276(7):555-560.

    29. Tschida, *op. cit.,* p. 25.

    30. Olmos, David R., and Michael A. Hiltzik. 1995, August 29. "Doctors' Authority, Pay Dwindle Under HMOs." *Los Angeles Times,* pp. A1, A10-A11; p. A10.

31. Reinhardt, Uwe. 1996, April. "Less Pay, No Less Worthwhile." *The New Physician,* pp. 5-6.

32. Krieger, *op. cit.*

33. Tschida, Molly, and Paul Jung. 1996, November. "Managed Care Strikes Again." *The New Physician,* p. 5.

34. *Front and Center, Leading the Health Professions into the Next Century* (The Center for the Health Professions, University of California, San Francisco). 1997, Spring, 1(3):1-8.

35. Tschida, *op. cit.,* p. 25.

36. Roan, Shari. 1997. "New Doctors Need HMO Training Panel Says." *Los Angeles Times,* pp. A1, A15-A16.

37. *Ibid.,* pp. A15-A16.

38. *Ibid.,* p. A15.

39. *Ibid.,* p. A15.

40. *Ibid.,* pp. A15-A16.

41. Ginzberg, Eli. 1996, April. "Time Will Tell." *The New Physician,* p. 8.

42. Reinhardt, *op. cit.,* p. 6.

43. Krieger, *op cit.*

44. Coombs, Robert H. 1997. *Drug-Impaired Professionals.* Cambridge, MA: Harvard University Press.

45. Roark, Anne C. 1990, April. "The Good Doctor." *Los Angeles Times,* pp. 24, 38.

46. Holmes, Oliver Wendell. 1949. "Temptation of Becoming Ground Flat." *Treasury of the Christian Faith.* New York: Association Press. Copyrighted by the National Board of Young Men's Christian Association, p. 740.

47. Tanner, Obert C. 1955. *Christ's Ideals for Living.* Salt Lake City, UT: Deseret Sunday School Board, p. 114.

48. Baruch, Bernard, cited in Richard L. Evans, 1961, July 9. "Balance, Moderation, Judgment." Radio broadcast titled *The Spoken Word,* KSL radio and the Columbia Broadcasting System, p. 656.

49. Campbell, Angus. 1981. *The Sense of Well-Being in America.* New York: McGraw-Hill, p. 73.

Index